THE ESSENTIAL ANTI-INFLAMMATORY PATHWAY

How to Restore Balance, Reverse Chronic Symptoms, and Unlock Lifelong Wellness through Nutrition

© 2024 by Autumn Bennett

All rights reserved. No part of this publication may be reproduced, distributed, or transmitted in any form or by any means, including photocopying, recording, or other electronic or mechanical methods, without the prior written permission of the publisher, except in the case of brief quotations embodied in critical reviews and certain other noncommercial uses permitted by copyright law.

TABLE OF CONTENT

INTRODUCTION 10

CHAPTER 1: WHAT YOU SHOULD KNOW ABOUT INFLAMMATION TRIGGERS? 16

CHAPTER 2: REVERSING AND CALMING INFLAMMATORY FLARE-UP 24

POTATOES, OATMEAL, EGGS AND OTHER BREAKFAST 32

SALADS, WRAPS AND LIGHT MEALS 55

VEGETARIAN AND VEGAN 85

SOUPS AND STEWS 123

MEAT, SEAFOOD, POULTRY AND OTHER PROTEINS 143

GRAINS AND LEGUMES 181

SMOOTHIES, TEAS AND BEVERAGES 200

30 DAYS MEAL PLAN

FLARE UP TRACKER

Beginner Anti Inflammatory Cook Starter Pack

Starting an anti-inflammatory diet might be stressful at first, particularly if you aren't used to cooking much. Don't worry, our starting pack will walk you through what to anticipate and include practical cooking suggestions to help you incorporate anti-inflammatory foods into your daily meals. You'll learn that cooking to decrease inflammation is more than simply what you can't eat; it's about embracing healthy, flavorful meals that help heal your body from inside.

What to Expect When Beginning an Anti-Inflammatory Diet

1. Initial Learning Curve: You'll most likely need to familiarize yourself with anti-inflammatory substances and recipes. If you're unfamiliar with specific spices, grains, or fruit, you may find yourself researching how to cook them or exploring shopping aisles with a more interested eye.

2. Simpler cookery Methods: Anti-inflammatory cookery often focuses on simple preparation techniques that highlight the natural tastes of entire foods. Instead of deep frying or heavy processing, expect to utilize roasting, steaming, and sautéing methods.

3. New Flavors and Textures: You will come across some unexpected ingredients, such as turmeric, quinoa, and leafy greens like arugula. This is a great opportunity to discover new tastes and sensations.

4. Feeling More Energized: When you start eating more anti-inflammatory foods, you may experience improvements in your energy levels, digestion, and general health. This is one of the primary motivators to keep going, even if the adjustment is difficult at first.

5. Meal Prep Can Be Your Best Friend: To succeed, expect to devote more time to meal planning and preparation, particularly if you're accustomed to convenience foods. Preparing quantities of cereals, veggies, and meats ahead of time can help you save time throughout the week.

Essential Cooking Tips for Anti-Inflammatory Beginners

1. Stock your pantry with key ingredients

Anti-inflammatory cooking begins with a well-stocked pantry. Here are some basics to have On hand.

- Healthy fats include extra virgin olive oil, avocado oil, and coconut oil. These fats are not only nutrient dense, but also anti-inflammatory.
- Spices and Herbs: Turmeric, ginger, garlic, cumin, cinnamon, rosemary, and thyme are crucial for taste and anti-inflammatory properties.
- Whole Grains: Brown rice, quinoa, buckwheat, and oats are all excellent alternatives to processed grains. They are abundant in fiber and minerals that help reduce inflammation.
- Nuts and Seeds: Almonds, walnuts, chia seeds, and flaxseeds are high in omega-3 fatty acids, which are beneficial in lowering inflammation.
- Legumes: Beans and lentils are high in fiber and plant-based protein, making them an excellent complement to soups, salads, and side dishes.
- Leafy Greens: Stock up on spinach, kale, arugula, and collard greens. They're simple to include into smoothies, salads, and even stews.
- Berries: Blueberries, strawberries, and raspberries are antioxidant-rich and may be utilized in a variety of recipes, including smoothies and salads.

2. Mastering Simple Cooking Techniques

Anti-inflammatory foods shine when cooked simply and healthfully. Here are the essentials you'll utilize most frequently:

- Roasting: Ideal for veggies like sweet potatoes, Brussels sprouts, carrots, and cauliflower. Roasting enhances the natural sweetness of vegetables without using much oil.

Tip: Toss veggies with olive oil, salt, pepper, and turmeric before roasting for 20-30 minutes at 400°F (200°C).

- Sautéing: To swiftly sauté leafy greens, garlic, onions, and spices, heat a tiny quantity of olive oil. This approach is ideal for stir-fries or fast side dishes.

Tip: Sauté veggies with garlic and ginger over medium heat for a blast of anti-inflammatory flavor.

- Steaming is great for keeping nutrients in veggies, especially greens like broccoli or kale. Steaming is fast and needs no additional fat.

Tip: After steaming, sprinkle with lemon juice and olive oil for extra flavor.

- Blending: Anti-inflammatory smoothies and soups are an excellent method to get nutrients. Use a high-powered blender to combine fruits, leafy greens, and anti-inflammatory ingredients such as turmeric or ginger.

Tip: For an invigorating start to the day, make a Turmeric-Ginger Smoothie with frozen pineapple, a pinch of turmeric, fresh ginger, almond milk, and spinach.

3: Make Batch Cooking Your Best Friend

Cooking in bulk is essential for decreasing your everyday time spent in the kitchen. Here are some tips for preparing in advance:

- Cook Grains: Make a big quantity of quinoa, brown rice, or buckwheat and refrigerate for usage throughout the week. These grains create a great basis for salads, bowls, and sides.

Tip: Cooked grains may be stored in an airtight container for up to four days.

- Roast veggies: Roast a large tray of mixed veggies (e.g., sweet potatoes, carrots, cauliflower, and Brussels sprouts) to serve as a side dish or put into salad.

Batch Cook Protein: Prepare the week's chicken breasts, salmon filets, or tofu by baking or grilling them. To keep meals interesting, try pairing them with various sauces and sides.
Tip: To add variety, season proteins with olive oil, herbs, and lemon juice.

4. Spice It Up for Maximum Results

Spices are your hidden weapon for anti-inflammatory cooking. Turmeric, in example, is well-known for its anti-inflammatory qualities, but it may have a harsh flavor if you aren't accustomed to it.

- Turmeric: Mix it with black pepper to increase its absorption in the body. Add turmeric to soups, smoothies, and roasted veggies.

- Ginger: Fresh ginger provides zest and warmth to both savory and sweet meals. It works well in stir-fries, marinades, and even shredded into drinks.
- Cayenne Pepper: If you like heat, cayenne is a strong anti-inflammatory spice that may be sprinkled over roasted vegetables or meats.

5. Focus on Flavor Boosting Techniques

Anti-inflammatory meals do not need to be bland. Here are some flavor-enhancing strategies to improve your meals:

- Use Fresh Herbs: Fresh herbs, such as cilantro, parsley, and mint, may quickly brighten a meal. Add them near the end of the cooking process to preserve their taste and nutrition.

- Make Simple Dressings: Making your own dressing may add excitement to any salad or grain bowl. Combine olive oil, lemon juice, garlic, and mustard to make a tart and anti-inflammatory sauce.

- Citrus Zest: Lemon or lime zest provides an exceptional depth of flavor without adding calories. It goes nicely with both protein and veggies.

Sample Beginner Recipe: Turmeric Roasted Sweet Potatoes

Ingredients: 2 medium sweet potatoes, peeled and cubed, 1 tbsp olive oil, 1 tsp powdered turmeric, and 1/2 tsp ground cumin.
- Add salt and pepper to taste.

Instructions:
1. Preheat your oven to 400°F (200°C).
2. In a large bowl, combine the sweet potato cubes, olive oil, turmeric, cumin, salt, and pepper.
3. Place the potatoes in a single layer on a baking sheet lined with parchment paper.
4. Roast for 25–30 minutes, turning halfway through, until golden and crispy.
5. Serve as a side dish or combine with a salad for an added anti-inflammatory benefit.

With these ideas, you'll be well on your way to understanding the fundamentals of anti-inflammatory cooking. Start small, experiment with new ingredients, and prioritize simple, delectable meals that feed both your body and mind. As you go, you'll discover that it's not only about the dishes you're trying, but also about how these meals make you feel better day after day.

INTRODUCTION

Every day, millions of individuals inadvertently feed the fires of inflammation via the foods they consume. Chronic inflammation has become a hidden pandemic, leading to an increase in significant health disorders such as heart disease, diabetes, arthritis, and even cancer. Recent research indicates that the traditional Western diet, which is high in processed foods, sweets, and bad fats, contributes significantly to this persistent inflammation. Many individuals are unaware that, although inflammation is a normal defensive mechanism, it may cause damage to healthy cells, tissues, and organs over time, leading to long-term health concerns.

According to the World Health Organization, non-communicable diseases (NCDs) now account for approximately 71% of all worldwide deaths, with chronic inflammation induced by poor dietary choices being a major contributor. In fact, the National Institutes of Health has shown that diets high in refined carbohydrates, processed meats, and sugary drinks are major contributors to systemic inflammation. Despite this frightening trend, the food industry continues to produce highly processed, inflammatory items, leaving consumers mostly oblivious of the hazards hiding on their plates.

I have been there myself. For years, I struggled with inexplicable lethargy, joint discomfort, and periods of cognitive fog that hampered my everyday activities. I tried drugs, vitamins, and lifestyle modifications, but none provided long-term relief. It wasn't until I started researching the function of food in inflammation that I realized a crucial truth: the things we eat may either fuel or extinguish the fire of inflammation. That knowledge changed everything for me. I eventually started feeling better from inside after changing my diet to include more complete, nutrient-dense, anti-inflammatory foods.

This book was inspired by my personal experience and the urgent desire to share what I've learned with others. It is a resource for anybody looking to take charge of their health by lowering inflammation via eating. I'll guide you through the science of inflammation, explain how your food may either increase or decrease inflammation, and present practical, easy-to-follow recipes to help you fuel your body and regain equilibrium.

Whether you're coping with chronic sickness, weariness, or just wish to avoid future health issues, this book will teach you how to harness the healing power of food. With each mouthful, you can help your body's natural capacity to combat inflammation and regain its health.

What is inflammation?

Inflammation is the body's natural defense mechanism, a necessary component of the immune response that protects us against hazardous invaders such as germs, viruses, or trauma. In its most basic form, inflammation is the body's method of directing the immune system to repair damaged tissue or protect against invading substances. You've probably felt inflammation firsthand—consider the redness and swelling that happens when you cut your finger or twist your ankle. This is acute inflammation, and it indicates that your body is trying to cure itself.

In some instances, inflammation is both required and helpful. It is the body's method of directing immune cells, hormones, and nutrients to the area of damage or illness. Without inflammation, wounds would fester, infections would become fatal, and healing would not occur.

However, inflammation is a two-edged sword. While acute inflammation is a short-term healing process, chronic inflammation may cause issues if it lasts for weeks, months, or years. Chronic inflammation is more subtle and insidious, occurring at low levels all throughout the body. Instead of healing, chronic inflammation may cause long-term harm to tissues and organs, leading to a variety of disorders.

The Body's Immune Response and When Things Go Wrong

Understanding inflammation requires an understanding of the immune system. Our immune system is a complex network of cells, proteins, and organs that collaborate to protect against dangerous intruders such as pathogens (bacteria, viruses, and other foreign substances).

When the immune system identifies a danger, it initiates an inflammatory reaction, releasing immune cells and substances that isolate and destroy the invader or repair injured tissues.

The earliest symptoms of inflammation—heat, redness, swelling, and pain—are generated by increased blood flow and immunological activity in the afflicted region. The body is deploying its defenses. Once the danger has been eliminated, the inflammation goes down, and the immune system returns to its natural, balanced condition.

However, when things go wrong and the inflammatory response persists, it becomes chronic. Instead of providing a short-term solution, the immune system remains on high alert, producing inflammatory signals even when there is no genuine danger to combat. Over time, uncontrolled inflammation may harm healthy tissues, contribute to the development of autoimmune disorders, and pave the way for chronic illnesses such as heart disease, type 2 diabetes, and cancer.

Understanding the Differences between Acute and Chronic Inflammation

Acute inflammation

Acute inflammation is temporary and usually develops in reaction to an injury, illness, or other damaging event. For example, if you sprain your ankle, cut your hand, or get the flu, your body produces acute inflammation to facilitate recovery. This form of inflammation is very transitory and goes away as the body heals from the injury or illness. Common signs of acute inflammation are:

Symptoms may include redness, swelling, pain, heat, and temporary loss of function (similar to a sprained joint).

This form of inflammation is vital for healing and shows that the body is functioning properly.

Chronic inflammation

Chronic inflammation, on the other hand, is less noticeable and may linger for months or years. Instead of disappearing when the body heals, it lingers, and the immune system continues to transmit inflammatory signals. Chronic inflammation often occurs without any evident damage or illness and may be caused by long-term exposure to irritants such as smoking, a poor diet, or environmental contaminants. It may also be caused by autoimmune illnesses, in which the body erroneously targets healthy cells.

Chronic inflammation, unlike acute inflammation, does not produce visible symptoms. It often operates quietly, damaging cells and tissues from the inside out, gradually leading to the development of illnesses such as:

- Cardiovascular Disease: Chronic inflammation may damage arteries, causing atherosclerosis (plaque accumulation) and raising the risk of heart attacks and strokes.
- Type 2 Diabetes: Inflammation causes insulin resistance, which is a major factor in the development of diabetes.
- Cancer: Chronic inflammation may damage DNA and encourage tumor development.
- Autoimmune Diseases: Chronic inflammation causes conditions such as rheumatoid arthritis, lupus, and inflammatory bowel disease, in which the immune system misidentifies and targets healthy tissues.
- Alzheimer's disease: It is thought that chronic inflammation in the brain contributes to neurodegenerative disorders such as Alzheimer's.

The difference between acute and chronic inflammation is critical. While acute inflammation indicates that the body is defending itself against an immediate assault, persistent inflammation indicates that something is awry and may have major health repercussions.

How Chronic Inflammation Causes Disease

Inflammation that persists in the body produces broad cellular damage. Consider chronic inflammation to be a slow-burning fire within you that causes damage to whatever it touches. This continual state of immunological activity wears on the body over time and may harm healthy cells, tissues, and organs.

Here's how chronic inflammation affects some of the most prevalent diseases:

1. Heart Disease: Chronic inflammation is a key factor in the development of atherosclerosis, in which the walls of arteries harden with plaque. Over time, this plaque hardens and inhibits

blood flow, potentially leading to heart attacks or strokes. Inflammation also makes these plaques more susceptible to rupture, resulting in abrupt cardiovascular events.

2. Type 2 Diabetes: Inflammation may affect how the body reacts to insulin, the hormone that controls blood sugar. Over time, insulin resistance causes high blood sugar levels and, ultimately, diabetes. In fact, many persons with type 2 diabetes show signs of chronic inflammation.

3. Cancer: Chronic inflammation may aid in the development and progression of cancer. Inflammatory cells produce substances that may damage DNA and promote the creation of malignant cells. In certain circumstances, inflammation may promote tumor growth and spread.

4. Rheumatoid Arthritis: This autoimmune illness causes persistent inflammation in the joints. The immune system assaults the lining of the joints, causing discomfort, swelling, and ultimately joint destruction.

5. Alzheimer's Disease: Research has connected brain inflammation to neurodegenerative disorders such as Alzheimer's. Over time, this inflammation harms brain cells and leads to cognitive loss.

Chronic inflammation does more than only contribute to illness; it is often a driving force behind the onset and progression of various disorders. The good news is that by treating chronic inflammation via food and lifestyle changes, we may lower our chance of acquiring certain illnesses while also promoting the body's healing process.

Scientifically Proven Anti-Inflammatory Diet Benefits

Scientific study has repeatedly shown that what we consume may either increase or decrease inflammation. A diet high in anti-inflammatory foods protects against chronic illnesses and improves general well-being. Numerous studies have revealed that diets high in processed foods, sugar, and bad fats increase inflammation, while diets high in whole, nutrient-dense foods may help reduce inflammation.

The following are the known advantages of an anti-inflammatory diet:

1. Reduced Risk of Chronic Disease: Numerous studies have shown that persons who follow an anti-inflammatory diet are less likely to acquire heart disease, type 2 diabetes, and certain malignancies. The Mediterranean diet, which includes fruits, vegetables, whole grains, healthy fats, and lean meats, has been associated with decreased inflammation and a lower risk of heart disease and stroke.

2. Improved Digestive Health: Chronic inflammation may cause damage to the gut lining, resulting in illnesses such as irritable bowel syndrome (IBS) and inflammatory bowel disease. An anti-inflammatory diet promotes gut health by providing fiber, healthy fats, and nutrients that help balance the microbiota and protect the digestive system.

3. Better Joint Health: For those suffering from arthritis or joint pain, an anti-inflammatory diet may help decrease swelling and stiffness. Omega-3 fatty acids, found in fatty fish such as salmon, are very helpful in reducing joint inflammation.

4. Enhanced Brain Function: Anti-inflammatory foods, especially those high in antioxidants and omega-3s, have been demonstrated to promote brain health and lower the risk of neurodegenerative disorders such as Alzheimer's. Berries, leafy greens, and walnuts are all high in nutrients that benefit the brain.

5. Weight Management: Chronic inflammation is often related to obesity. Reduced inflammation by food makes weight management simpler, since inflammation relates to insulin resistance and metabolic diseases. Anti-inflammatory meals such as whole grains, lean meats, and vegetables aid with weight management by increasing metabolism and decreasing cravings for processed, inflammatory foods.

6. Improved Mood and Mental Health: A growing body of research has linked inflammation to mental health issues such as sadness and anxiety. Diets that lower inflammation may benefit mental health by promoting emotional well-being and cognitive performance.

Chronic inflammation is at the basis of many contemporary health issues, but we have the capacity to prevent it—specifically, via the foods we consume. An anti-inflammatory diet is more than a fad; it's a scientifically proven strategy to feed the body, lower illness risk, and promote recovery.

1: WHAT YOU SHOULD KNOW ABOUT INFLAMMATION TRIGGERS

To properly control and eliminate inflammation in the body, we must first identify the factors that cause it. While inflammation may be induced by a variety of variables, one of the most important is our diet. Beyond nutrition, our contemporary lives and surroundings also contribute significantly to inflammation.

Foods that promote inflammation

One of the key causes of chronic inflammation is the contemporary diet, particularly the abundance of highly processed and refined foods. These foods often include substances that, when ingested on a regular basis, cause the body to produce a prolonged inflammatory response. Let's look at a few of the most prevalent inflammatory foods.

1. Processed sugars

Sugar is one of the most inflammatory components in today's diet. It may be found not just in sweets like candies, cakes, and cookies, but also in processed foods such as sauces, salad dressings, and even bread. When we ingest sugar, our blood glucose levels rise, prompting the body to produce insulin. Repeated sugar surges cause insulin resistance and inflammation, which may contribute to obesity, type 2 diabetes, and cardiovascular disease.

Foods rich in processed sugar include soda and sugary beverages.
- packaged food, such as cookies, cakes, and pastries.
- Candy & chocolates.
- Sweetened cereals and granola bars.

2. Refined Carbs

Refined carbohydrates, such as white bread, white rice, and pasta, are stripped of fiber and minerals during processing, leaving just simple carbs that the body rapidly turns to sugar. Refined carbohydrates, like processed sugars, promote blood sugar increases and contribute to the inflammatory response. A diet heavy in refined carbohydrates may eventually lead to insulin resistance and an increased risk of chronic illnesses such as diabetes and heart disease.

Common sources of refined carbs are white bread and buns.
- Pasta prepared with white flour
- White rice.
- Pastries and other products prepared with refined flour.

3. Trans Fats

Trans fats are one of the most inflammatory fats. They are present in partly hydrogenated oils, which are often used in processed and fried meals to improve shelf life. Trans fats not only cause inflammation, but they also raise LDL (bad) cholesterol while decreasing HDL (good) cholesterol, increasing the risk of heart disease and other inflammatory disorders.

Cuisine with trans fats include fried and quick cuisine.
- Packaged snacks, such as chips and crackers.
- Margarine with Shortening
- Commercially prepared products such as pies, cookies, and cakes

4. Red and processed meats

While meat may be part of a healthy diet, some forms of meat, particularly processed meats, have been shown to increase inflammation. Processed meats such as bacon, sausage, hot dogs, and deli meats are often rich in preservatives, nitrates, and other substances that promote inflammation. Furthermore, red meat, especially when ingested in big amounts, has been associated with elevated levels of inflammatory markers in the body. Red meat contains chemicals such as advanced glycation end products (AGEs) and arachidonic acid, which are thought to cause inflammation.

Examples of inflammatory meats include bacon, sausage, and hot dogs.
- Deli meats, including ham and salami

- Beef and pork, especially fatty slices.

5. Dairy Products

Consuming dairy products may cause an inflammatory reaction in certain individuals, particularly those who are lactose intolerant or sensitive to dairy. Dairy may induce gastrointestinal irritation, which may lead to inflammation in the stomach and elsewhere. Even for people who do not have lactose intolerance, full-fat dairy products are heavy in saturated fats, which may cause inflammation when ingested in excess.

Inflammatory dairy products include whole milk and cream.
- Cheese, particularly processed versions.
Butter with ice cream.
- Yogurt with additional sugar.

6. Alcohol

Excessive alcohol use is another major inflammatory factor. Alcohol may irritate the intestinal lining and disturb the balance of good microorganisms in the gut, causing inflammation. Over time, alcohol may also cause liver inflammation and damage, raising the risk of chronic illnesses such as liver disease.

While moderate alcohol use (such as a glass of red wine) has been associated with certain health advantages, frequent or excessive drinking should be avoided if you want to minimize inflammation.

Hidden Inflammatory Triggers in Common Diets

While the obvious causes, such as sugar, trans fats, and processed meats, are widely recognized, many popular diets include other inflammatory triggers. These triggers might be modest, but they nevertheless contribute to chronic inflammation if ingested on a regular basis.

1. Gluten

Gluten is a protein present in wheat, barley, and rye. While celiac disease affects a tiny fraction of the population, many individuals have gluten sensitivities or intolerances, which may cause digestive problems and inflammation. Consuming gluten may activate an immunological response that produces gut inflammation, resulting in symptoms such as bloating, diarrhea, and exhaustion.

Gluten is often found in wheat products such as bread, pasta, and cereals.
- Baked products, including cakes, cookies, and pastries
- Beer and other malt drinks.

2. Artificial additives and preservatives

Many packaged and processed meals include artificial chemicals, preservatives, and colorings that may trigger inflammation. Ingredients such as monosodium glutamate (MSG), artificial sweeteners, and high-fructose corn syrup have all been related to increased inflammation in the body. These chemicals disturb the gut microbiota, causing an imbalance in beneficial bacteria and raising the risk of inflammation.

Watch out for these ingredients in packaged foods.
- Frozen dinners.
- Fast food.
- Sweetened drinks.

3. Omega 6 Fatty Acids

While certain fats are helpful, omega-6 fatty acids, present in many vegetable oils, may cause inflammation if ingested in excess. These oils are often utilized in processed and fried meals, and although the body requires certain omega-6 fatty acids, a balance of omega-6 and omega-3 fatty acids is essential. A diet heavy in omega-6 and deficient in omega-3 may cause inflammation.

Sources of omega-6 fatty acids include corn oil, soybean oil, and sunflower oil.
- Processed snack foods.
- Fried food.

4. Hidden sugars

Sugar is not just present in candies and pastries. It's buried in a variety of meals, even many we wouldn't normally consider "sweet." Foods like store-bought sauces, condiments, and salad dressings sometimes have added sugars, which may cause inflammation. Many "healthy" goods, such as flavored yogurt, granola bars, and fruit juices, contain hidden sugars, making it simple to eat more than you think.

Be aware of hidden sugars in
- Store-bought pasta sauces.
- BBQ sauce and ketchup.
- Fruit-flavored yogurts
- Sports beverages and flavored water.

Environmental and Lifestyle Triggers

Inflammation is impacted not just by what you consume, but also by your surroundings and lifestyle. Stress, a lack of sleep, and exposure to environmental pollutants are all risk factors for chronic inflammation.

1. Stress

Stress is a primary cause of inflammation in the body. When we are stressed, the body produces cortisol, a hormone that, in tiny doses, helps control the immune system. However, persistent stress causes extended cortisol release, which may inhibit the immune system and trigger an inflammatory response. Long-term stress has been related to heart disease, depression, and autoimmune illnesses, all of which are affected by inflammation.

2. Lack of sleep

Sleep is essential for good health, and a lack of it impairs the body's capacity to manage inflammation. Chronic sleep deprivation raises levels of inflammatory indicators such as C-reactive protein, which is linked to an increased risk of heart disease and other inflammatory disorders. Getting 7-9 hours of sleep per night is essential for lowering inflammation and improving overall health.

3. The Sedentary Lifestyle

A lack of physical exercise might lead to chronic inflammation. Regular exercise reduces inflammation by reducing the body's pro-inflammatory chemicals. A sedentary lifestyle, defined by prolonged sitting or inactivity, may raise the risk of obesity, insulin resistance, and chronic inflammation.

4. Smoking

Smoking is one of the most powerful inflammatory triggers. The chemicals in cigarette smoke cause direct damage to the lungs and blood vessels, resulting in inflammation. Smoking also raises the body's free radical levels, which contribute to oxidative stress and inflammation, raising the risk of heart disease, cancer, and respiratory disorders.

Environmental Toxins' Inflammatory Effects

Aside from nutrition and lifestyle, the environment we live in might cause inflammation via exposure to numerous chemicals. These poisons may be found in the air we breathe, the water we drink, and even the goods we use every day.

1. Air pollution

Pollution, particularly in metropolitan areas, is a major cause of inflammation. Exposure to airborne contaminants such as particulate matter (PM) from car emissions, industrial activities, and smoking may cause inflammation in the lungs and throughout the body. Long-term exposure to air pollution has been related to an increased risk of asthma, lung illness, and cardiovascular problems.

2. Heavy Metal

Heavy metals such as lead, mercury, and cadmium may build in the body, causing chronic inflammation. These metals are present in polluted water, some seafood, and even some home items. Over time, heavy metal exposure may harm tissues and organs, causing inflammation and raising the risk of illnesses such as renal disease and neurological problems.

3. Pesticides and Chemicals

Pesticides and chemicals in our food, water, and home items may potentially cause inflammation. Many pesticides used in agriculture have been shown to have detrimental effects on the body, and long-term exposure, even in little doses, may result in the buildup of dangerous compounds that contribute to chronic inflammation. These substances alter the body's normal equilibrium and may influence the endocrine and immunological systems, causing an increased inflammatory response.

Chemicals in cleaning goods, cosmetics, and even plastics (such as BPA and phthalates) all add to the body's toxic load. Over time, these poisons may build, particularly in the liver and fat cells, causing persistent inflammation. This is why limiting exposure to environmental pollutants is an important part of controlling chronic inflammation.

Practical Steps to Reduce Your Exposure to Environmental Toxins

While it is hard to eradicate all environmental toxins, there are actions you can do to limit your exposure and diminish the inflammatory effects on your body.

1. Choose Organic Foods

Organic foods are cultivated without the use of synthetic pesticides and fertilizers, making them a safer alternative for limiting exposure to dangerous chemicals. While organic food might be more costly, concentrating on the "Dirty Dozen" (fruits and vegetables with the highest pesticide levels) can help you decide which things to purchase organic.

2. Filter your water

Many tap water sources include small levels of heavy metals, chlorine, and other pollutants, which may cause irritation over time. Installing a high-quality water filter for your drinking water and shower will help decrease your exposure to these dangerous chemicals.

3. Use non-toxic cleaning products

Switching to natural cleaning solutions made with vinegar, baking soda, and essential oils will drastically limit your exposure to harmful chemicals. Avoid cleansers containing strong artificial smells and substances such as ammonia or bleach, which may irritate the respiratory system and cause irritation.

4: Limit Plastic Use

Avoid using plastic containers, particularly for food storage and cooking, since they may leach chemicals such as BPA into your food. Choose glass, stainless steel, or silicone wherever feasible. If you must use plastic, avoid heating it since this might enhance the release of hazardous chemicals.

5. Increase Indoor Air Quality

Because we spend so much time inside, your home's air quality may have a significant impact on your total exposure to contaminants. Simple efforts such as utilizing an air purifier, frequently ventilating your house, and introducing indoor plants that naturally filter the air (such as spider plants and peace lilies) may all help minimize airborne contaminants that cause inflammation.

6. Reduce Exposure to Heavy Metals

Be careful about the seafood you consume, since bigger species, such as tuna and swordfish, are more likely to contain mercury. Instead, choose for smaller fish, such as sardines and salmon, which are lower in toxins. Also, check for any municipal water warnings on lead or other heavy metals in your area, and consider utilizing a water filter system if necessary.

Chronic inflammation is at the basis of many contemporary illnesses, but by understanding these triggers and implementing modest dietary, lifestyle, and environmental modifications, you may drastically lower your inflammatory burden.

The good news is that it is never too late to implement these adjustments. Small changes, such as replacing processed meals with full, natural components, purchasing organic produce wherever feasible, and avoiding exposure to environmental contaminants, may contribute to significant gains in your health over time. And remember that lowering inflammation is a marathon, not a sprint. Every good decision you make moves you closer to a better, more balanced existence.

2: REVERSING AND CALMING INFLAMMATORY FLARE-UP

If you're experiencing an inflammatory flare-up, don't worry—you can take actions to reduce inflammation and start the healing process. Let's look at how you may reverse and control inflammation using an elimination diet, stress management methods like Yoga Nidra, safe supplements, and the advantages of exercise.

The Inflammation Elimination Diet Plan

An elimination diet is one of the most efficient methods for reducing inflammation in the body. This sort of diet entails avoiding items known to cause inflammation for a period of time before gradually adding them to determine which ones are causing your symptoms. The idea is to identify and remove particular foods that cause inflammation in your body.

Here's how to do an inflammatory elimination diet:

1. Begin by eliminating common inflammatory foods:
For 2 to 4 weeks, avoid eating items that are known to cause inflammation. This includes:
- Processed foods (packaged snacks; fast food)
- Sugar and artificial sweeteners.
- Refined carbs (white bread and pastries)
- Trans fats and hydrogenated oils (common in fried meals)
- Dairy goods (for those sensitive to casein or lactose)
- Gluten-containing grains (wheat, barley, and rye).
- Red meat and processed meats (such as sausages and bacon).
- Alcohol

2. Focus on anti-inflammatory foods:
While you're removing inflammatory foods, replace them with complete, nutrient-dense, anti-inflammatory alternatives. Include:

- Leafy greens: spinach, kale, and arugula.
- Fatty fish: Salmon, sardines, and mackerel (high in omega-3 fatty acids).
- Berries: Blueberries, strawberries, and raspberries (high in antioxidants).
- Nuts and seeds: Almonds, walnuts, flaxseeds, chia seed
- Turmeric and ginger: Both have powerful anti-inflammatory properties
- Olive oil is a heart-healthy lipid that helps decrease inflammation.
- Herbal teas: Chamomile and green tea.

3. Reintroduce Foods:

Following the elimination phase, gradually reintroduce the deleted foods, leaving a 2-3 day interval between each reintroduction. Pay particular attention to how your body reacts—any bloating, headaches, joint pain, or other inflammatory symptoms may suggest that you are sensitive to that meal.

This technique will assist you in developing a specific anti-inflammatory diet that is most effective for your body. It's worth noting that removing too many food categories without sufficient preparation might lead to nutritional deficits, so consulting with a nutritionist may be beneficial.

Stress Management for Inflammatory Control

During the course of writing this book, I got helpful stress management advice from a professional who provided a unique viewpoint on how we often misinterpret and mismanage stress. This understanding changed my perspective on coping with life's challenges, and I hope it does the same for you.

Stress is more than simply a feeling or a passing mood that may be alleviated with quick treatments like yoga, squeezing a stress ball, or working out. It is a physical response in the body indicating that something is wrong and must be addressed. We often confuse stress for a sensation and concentrate on things that make us feel better momentarily, rather than addressing the underlying problem.

Consider stress to be a kind of financial debt; just feeling better about your money is insufficient; you must also take concrete efforts to balance your budget. Similarly, stress accumulates in your life as bricks stack on a graph. Everyone has a specific stress threshold, and when the pressures in your life become too many, they might drive you over that barrier, possibly leading to burnout or despair. Depression, in this view, is your body's method of shutting down when overwhelmed, similar to how a body protects essential organs when freezing to death.

So, how do you really handle stress? You eliminate stresses from your life. The idea is to make a mental or physical list of everything that is stressing you out, from little activities like replacing a lightbulb to major worries like preparing for an important meeting. Once you've prepared your list, begin addressing the items you can immediately. Each work you finish truly lightens your burden and relieves stress.

We often fool ourselves into believing we are lowering stress by participating in things that make us feel good, but these activities do not address the underlying reasons. Real stress management is determining what is weighing on you and gradually reducing those stressors. This method results in a more productive life and a clearer mind.

1. Stress Types: 1. Residual Stress (Emotional Baggage): These are pressures from the past—things you can't alter, such as childhood trauma or prior failures—that stick with you and influence your current state. While they are impossible to remove, understanding their existence allows you to handle them better.
2. Recurrent stress: These are routine duties that occur on a regular basis, such as bill payment or house maintenance. While they may seem little at first, they accumulate over time and may have a significant impact on your total stress load if not addressed regularly.
3. Time Sensitive Stress: These stresses loom in the future, such as a job interview or an impending deadline. Although you cannot address them immediately, you may mitigate their influence by being busy in the meantime, doing modest chores that will help clear the way when the time comes.

This stress management approach focuses on long-term solutions that address the root causes of stress in your life, rather than short fixes. Recognizing the underlying nature of stress and actively decreasing the obstacles can prepare you to deal with life's stresses and avoid burnout.

Here are some extra useful suggestions for stress management beyond simply addressing your problems head-on:

I. Identify your stress relievers: Take some time to determine which hobbies actually assist to ease your tension. It might be as easy as taking a hot bath, going on a walk in nature, listening to birds sing, or looking up at the stars. Perhaps it's something more strenuous, such as punching a bag or jogging a few kilometers. Once you've found these activities, make them a regular part of your routine. Build them into your daily routine and look forward to them as times of relaxation and comfort.

II. Include Physical Activity: Make sure that some of your stress relievers include physical activity. Exercise not only reduces stress by generating endorphins, but it also benefits your general health and fitness. Physical exercise, whether running, cycling, hiking, or boxing, helps to clear your mind and gives practical advantages that can be measured and seen. The idea is to discover something that resonates with you and really commit to it.

III. Develop a talent: Another way to reduce stress is to concentrate on activities that enable you to learn a new talent. Painting, for example, provides a creative outlet while simultaneously helping you develop a skill. Engaging in skill-building activities offers your mind something useful to concentrate on while also providing a feeling of achievement, which can be quite soothing.

IV. Leverage Nature: Spending time in nature is one of the most effective ways to reduce stress. Nature has a way of relaxing the mind, whether you're walking in the countryside, climbing a mountain, or just resting by a serene lake. Fresh air, natural sceneries, and physical exercise work together to reset your mental state and let you return to life with a revitalized feeling of clarity and peace. When stress becomes overpowering, walking outside may do wonders.

V. Consciously Focus on the Benefits: Whatever stress-relieving hobbies you pick, concentrate on how they benefit you. Don't simply go through the motions; recognize how the activity helps you feel better and immerse yourself in the experience. Whether you're racing through a 10k race or relaxing on a stroll, being present in the moment increases the stress-relieving benefits.

Identifying and truly interacting with your individual stress relievers allows you to properly manage and decrease stress in a sustained and highly personal manner.

Yoga Nidra for Stress Management

Chronic stress is one of the leading causes of inflammation in the body, and stress management is critical to reducing inflammatory flare-ups. While there are other stress management strategies available, one especially helpful practice is Yoga Nidra, often known as "yogic sleep."

Yoga Nidra is a guided meditation technique that leads you to the border of sleep while keeping you attentive and aware. It is a very calming technique that may help decrease stress hormones, soothe the neurological system, and reduce inflammation. This is how it works.

1. What to expect in a session:

A typical Yoga Nidra session involves lying down in a comfortable posture, closing your eyes, and listening to a guided meditation. The technique often includes a body scan, in which you mentally concentrate on various regions of your body and gradually relax each one.

2. Inflammation Benefits:
- Lowers Cortisol Levels High levels of the stress hormone cortisol have been related to chronic inflammation. Yoga Nidra helps to decrease cortisol, which reduces inflammation.
- Increases Relaxation: Yoga Nidra stimulates the parasympathetic nerve system, which controls the body's "rest and digest" response. This reduces the effects of stress and regulates the body's inflammatory response.
- Supports Better Sleep: Poor sleep might worsen inflammation. Yoga Nidra improves the quality of your sleep, which contributes to the body's healing process.

Follow (inflammationreset page on youtube for more on yoga nidra)

Regular Yoga Nidra practice may help relax both your mind and body, and it can be an effective therapy for reducing stress-induced inflammation.

Inflammatory Supplements That Are Safe to Use

While nutrition and stress management are essential for controlling inflammation, some supplements may also help to alleviate flare-ups. It's critical to choose supplements that are both safe and proven to have anti-inflammatory qualities. Here are a handful which research supports:

1. Omega-3 Fatty Acids (fish or algae oil):

Omega-3s are well-known for their anti-inflammatory effects. They assist in suppressing the production of inflammatory chemicals such as cytokines and prostaglandins. If you don't receive enough omega-3s from foods like fatty fish, fish oil or plant-based algal oil supplements are an excellent choice.

2. Curcumin (Turmeric Extract):

Curcumin is the primary ingredient in turmeric, and it has potent anti-inflammatory properties. However, curcumin is not readily absorbed by the body, hence it is often combined with black pepper extract (piperine) to improve absorption. For the greatest benefits, choose supplements that include both curcumin and piperine.

3. Ginger extract:

Ginger includes chemicals known as gingerols, which have anti-inflammatory and antioxidant activities. Ginger pills may help relieve pain and inflammation, especially in illnesses such as arthritis.

4. Probiotics:

A healthy gut microbiota is critical for regulating inflammation since an unbalanced gut may contribute to systemic inflammation. Probiotics assist to restore the balance of healthy bacteria in your stomach, which reduces inflammation and improves general immunity.

5. Vitamin D:

Vitamin D is required for immune system control, and low vitamin D levels have been linked to increased inflammation. If you're lacking in this vitamin, taking supplements may help decrease inflammation.

Before beginning any new supplements, contact your healthcare professional, particularly if you have pre-existing health concerns or are using medicines.

Exercise's Inflammation Control Benefits

Exercise is sometimes seen as a straightforward cure to a wide range of health issues, and the advantages of exercise in terms of inflammation are indisputable. Regular physical exercise is one of the most effective strategies to reduce inflammation since it improves both your body's inflammatory indicators and its overall immune response.

Here's how exercise may help you manage inflammation:

1. Reduces inflammation markers:

According to studies, regular exercise lowers levels of inflammatory indicators such as C-reactive protein (CRP) and cytokines. Chronic inflammation often results in higher levels of these markers.

2. Boosts circulation:

Exercise increases blood flow, which helps supply oxygen and nutrients to tissues while cleaning away toxins and waste items that may cause inflammation. This technique promotes speedier recovery and repair.

3. Helps Maintain a Healthy Weight

Maintaining a healthy weight is essential for reducing inflammation. Excess fat, particularly around the abdomen, produces pro-inflammatory compounds. Regular exercise helps you maintain a healthy weight and reduces inflammation.

4. Boosts endorphins and reduces stress:

Physical activity causes the release of endorphins, the body's natural mood boosters. Endorphins reduce stress, which is a major cause of chronic inflammation. Exercise can help control inflammation while also reducing stress.

5. Strengthens Immune System:

Moderate-intensity exercise improves immunological function, enabling the body to react more effectively to inflammation and infection. However, it is crucial to remember that excessive, high-intensity exercise may occasionally result in increased inflammation, so striking a balance is essential.

How to Use Exercise for Inflammation Control:

- Begin Slow: If you are new to exercising, start with low-impact activities such as walking, swimming, or cycling.
- Consistency is key: Aim for at least 30 minutes of moderate exercise five days a week. Even moderate exercises such as stretching or yoga might have anti-inflammatory properties.
- Mix It Up: To create a well-rounded regimen, combine aerobic workouts (such as jogging or brisk walking) with strength training (using weights or body resistance).
- Don't Forget Recovery: Give your body enough time to relax and recuperate, since over-exercising without proper rest may lead to inflammation.

POTATOES, OATMEAL, EGGS AND OTHER BREAKFAST

Tips:
- Prep ingredients like hard-boiled eggs and roasted potatoes in advance
- Keep frozen berries on hand
- Stock anti-inflammatory spices like turmeric, ginger, and cinnamon
- Consider making larger batches of bases (oatmeal, quinoa, potatoes) to use throughout the week

Sweet Potato Hash

Prep Time: 10 minutes

Cook Time: 25 minutes

Serving Size: 1 cup (makes 4 servings)

(Per 1-Cup Serving):

Calories: 175

Carbs: 30g

Sugar: 7g

Protein: 3g

Fat: 5g

2 medium sweet potatoes, peeled and diced about 4 cups

1 tablespoon olive oil

1 small red onion, finely chopped about 1/2 cup

1 bell pepper (any color), diced about 1 cup

2 cups fresh spinach, roughly chopped

2 cloves garlic, minced

1 teaspoon ground turmeric

1/2 teaspoon paprika

1/4 teaspoon ground cumin

Salt and black pepper to taste

Fresh parsley for garnish

Heat a large pan over medium heat and add the olive oil. Once heated, add the diced sweet potatoes. Cook for 10–12 minutes, stirring periodically, until the sweet potatoes soften and become golden brown.

In the skillet, combine the chopped red onion, bell pepper, and garlic. Sauté the onions and peppers for approximately 5-7 minutes, or until soft and tender.

Combine ground turmeric, paprika, cumin, salt, and black pepper. Mix well to evenly coat the sweet potatoes and veggies.

Cook the spinach in the pan for an additional 2-3 minutes, or until wilted.

Remove from the heat and garnish with fresh parsley, if preferred. Serve. Each serving is roughly one cup.

Overnight Oats

Prep Time: 5 minutes

Chill Time: 4 hours (or overnight)

Serving Size: 1 cup (makes 2 servings)

(Per 1-Cup Serving):

Calories: 250

Carbs: 35g

Sugar: 7g

Protein: 7g

Fat: 8g

- 1 cup rolled oats
- 1 cup unsweetened almond milk
- 1/2 cup plain coconut yogurt
- 1 tablespoon chia seeds
- 1 teaspoon ground turmeric
- 1/2 teaspoon ground cinnamon
- 1/4 teaspoon ground ginger
- 1 tablespoon maple syrup
- 1/2 teaspoon vanilla extract
- Fresh berries or nuts for topping

In a mixing bowl, combine the rolled oats, almond milk, coconut yogurt, chia seeds, turmeric, cinnamon, ginger, maple syrup, and vanilla extract. Stir well to mix.

Place the mixture in an airtight container or two jars and refrigerate for at least 4 hours, ideally overnight, to enable the oats to soak up the liquid and become creamy.

In the morning, give the oats a good stir, and if they are too thick, add a little more almond milk to get the appropriate consistency. Serve cold or warm, with optional fresh berries or nuts on top. Each serving is about 1 cup..

Egg Bowl

Prep Time: 10 minutes

Cook Time: 10 minutes

Serving Size: 1 bowl (makes 2 servings)

(Per Bowl):

Calories: 320

Carbs: 9g

Sugar: 2g

Protein: 14g

Fat: 26g

- 4 large eggs
- 1 tablespoon olive oil
- 2 cups baby spinach, roughly chopped
- 1 small avocado, diced
- 1/2 cup cherry tomatoes, halved
- 1/4 teaspoon ground turmeric
- 1/4 teaspoon paprika
- Salt and pepper to taste
- Fresh cilantro for garnish

Heat a little quantity of olive oil in a nonstick pan over medium heat. Crack the eggs into the pan, season with turmeric, paprika, salt, and pepper, and cook until sunny side up or scrambled (approximately 4-5 minutes).

In a separate small pan, heat the remaining olive oil over medium heat. Sauté the chopped spinach for 2-3 minutes, until wilted. Season gently with salt and pepper.

Divide the sautéed spinach into two dishes. Top each with two eggs, half of the chopped avocado, and a handful of cherry tomato halves.

For extra flavor, sprinkle with fresh cilantro and serve.

Potato Breakfast Bowl

Prep Time: 10 minutes

Cook Time: 20 minutes

Serving Size: 1 bowl (makes 2 servings)

(Per Bowl):

Calories: 350

Carbs: 25g

Sugar: 4g

Protein: 14g

Fat: 24g

2 medium purple potatoes, diced (about 2 cups)

1 tablespoon olive oil

1 small red onion, finely chopped (about 1/2 cup)

1/2 teaspoon ground turmeric

1/4 teaspoon paprika

4 large eggs

1/2 avocado, sliced

1/4 cup crumbled goat cheese

Salt and pepper to taste

Fresh parsley for garnish

In a large skillet, heat olive oil over medium heat. Cook the diced purple potatoes for 10-12 minutes, stirring regularly, until soft and slightly crunchy.

Cook the chopped red onion in the pan with the potatoes for another 5 minutes, or until the onions soften. Stir in the turmeric, paprika, salt, and pepper.

In a separate pan, prepare the eggs to your preference (sunny side up, scrambled, or poached).

Divide the cooked purple potatoes and onions into two dishes. Top with two eggs, half an avocado, and optional crumbled goat cheese.

Garnish with fresh parsley and serve

Ginger-Spiced Oatmeal

Prep Time: 5 minutes

Cook Time: 10 minutes

Serving Size: 1 cup (makes 2 servings)

(Per 1-Cup Serving):

Calories: 220

Carbs: 38g

Sugar: 7g

Protein: 6g

Fat: 5g

1 cup rolled oats

2 cups unsweetened almond milk

1 tablespoon fresh ginger, grated

1/2 teaspoon ground cinnamon

1 tablespoon maple syrup (optional)

1/4 teaspoon ground nutmeg

1/2 teaspoon vanilla extract

Fresh fruit (sliced bananas or berries) and nuts for topping

In a medium saucepan, mix the rolled oats, almond milk, fresh ginger, cinnamon, nutmeg, and maple syrup (optional). Bring the mixture to a simmer over medium heat.

Cook for 5-7 minutes, stirring regularly, until the oats are cooked and the mixture reaches the desired consistency.

Once the oats are completely cooked, stir in the vanilla essence.

Divide the oats into two dishes, approximately 1 cup each, and top with fresh fruit and nuts, if preferred.

Mediterranean Breakfast Plate

Prep Time: 10 minutes

Cook Time: 10 minutes

Serving Size: 1 plate (makes 2 servings)

4 large eggs

1 tablespoon olive oil

1/2 cup cherry tomatoes, halved

1/2 cucumber, sliced

1/4 cup Kalamata olives, pitted

1/2 avocado, sliced

1/4 cup hummus

1/4 cup crumbled feta cheese

Salt and pepper to taste

Fresh parsley for garnish

(Per Plate):

Calories: 370

Carbs: 15g

Sugar: 4g

Protein: 14g

Fat: 29g

Heat the olive oil in a nonstick pan over medium heat. Cook the eggs, either sunny-side up or scrambled, for around 4-5 minutes. Season with salt and pepper.

On each dish, lay two eggs, cherry tomatoes, cucumber slices, Kalamata olives, avocado slices, and a dab of hummus.

If desired, sprinkle each dish with crumbled feta cheese and garnish with fresh parsley.

Garnish with olive oil if preferred.

Berry-Loaded Quinoa Bowl

Prep Time: 5 minutes

Cook Time: 15 minutes

Serving Size: 1 bowl (makes 2 servings)

(Per Bowl):

Calories: 300

Carbs: 40g

Sugar: 10g

Protein: 9g

Fat: 11g

- 1/2 cup quinoa, rinsed
- 1 cup unsweetened almond milk
- 1 tablespoon maple syrup
- 1/2 teaspoon vanilla extract
- 1/2 cup mixed berries (blueberries, strawberries, raspberries)
- 1 tablespoon chia seeds
- 1/4 cup slivered almonds or walnuts
- Fresh mint for garnish

In a small saucepan, mix the quinoa and almond milk. Bring to a boil, then decrease heat to low, cover, and cook for 12-15 minutes, or until the quinoa is cooked and has absorbed the majority of the liquid.

Once cooked, add the maple syrup (if using) and vanilla essence.

Divide the cooked quinoa into two dishes. Top with mixed berries, chia seeds, and slivered almonds or walnuts, if preferred.

Garnish with fresh mint and serve right away..

Turmeric Potato Scramble

Prep Time: 10 minutes

Cook Time: 15 minutes

Serving Size: 1 bowl (makes 2 servings)

2 medium potatoes, diced (about 2 cups)

1 tablespoon olive oil

4 large eggs

(Per Bowl):

1/2 teaspoon ground turmeric

Calories: 320

1/4 teaspoon paprika

Carbs: 25g

Sugar: 3g

Protein: 14g

Fat: 18g

1 small red onion, chopped (about 1/2 cup)

1 cup baby spinach, roughly chopped

Salt and pepper to taste

Fresh parsley for garnish

Heat the olive oil in a large pan over medium heat. Cook the diced potatoes for 10-12 minutes, stirring regularly, until golden brown and soft.

Combine the chopped red onion, turmeric, paprika, salt, and pepper. Cook for 2-3 minutes, until the onions have softened.

Push the potato mixture to one side of the pan, then break the eggs into the open area. Scramble the eggs for approximately 2-3 minutes, then stir them into the potato mixture.

Stir in the chopped spinach and simmer for 1 minute, or until wilted.

Divide the scramble into two servings and top with fresh parsley, if preferred.

Toast

Prep Time: 5 minutes

Cook Time: 5 minutes

Serving Size: 1 slice (makes 2 servings)

(Per Slice):

Calories: 210

Carbs: 26g

Sugar: 2g

Protein: 4g

Fat: 10g

- 2 slices whole-grain or gluten-free bread
- 1/2 avocado, mashed
- 1/2 teaspoon ground turmeric
- 1/4 teaspoon red pepper flakes
- 1 tablespoon olive oil
- 1/4 cup cherry tomatoes, halved
- Salt and pepper to taste
- Fresh basil or parsley for garnish

Place the pieces of bread in a toaster or pan and toast until golden brown and crispy.

In a small bowl, mash the avocado and add the ground turmeric, salt, pepper, and red pepper flakes (if using).

Distribute the turmeric avocado mixture equally on each piece of toasted bread.

Top with halved cherry tomatoes and sprinkle with olive oil.

If wanted, garnish with fresh basil or parsley, then serve.

Cinnamon Apple Oatmeal

Prep Time: 5 minutes

Cook Time: 10 minutes

Serving Size: 1 bowl (makes 2 servings)

(Per Bowl):

Calories: 290

Carbs: 50g

Sugar: 12g

Protein: 6g

Fat: 7g

- 1 cup rolled oats
- 2 cups water or unsweetened almond milk
- 1 medium apple, diced (about 1 cup)
- 1 teaspoon ground cinnamon
- 1 tablespoon maple syrup
- 1/4 teaspoon salt
- 1 tablespoon walnuts or pecans, chopped
- Fresh apple slices and additional cinnamon for topping

In a medium saucepan, mix together rolled oats, water or almond milk, sliced apple, cinnamon, and salt. Bring to a boil over medium heat.

Once boiling, lower to a low heat and cook for 5-7 minutes, stirring periodically, until the oats are soft and have absorbed the majority of the liquid.

If using, stir in maple syrup and combine well.

Divide the oatmeal between two dishes. Top with chopped walnuts or pecans, fresh apple slices, and an additional sprinkling of cinnamon, if preferred.

Sweet Potato Toast

Prep Time: 5 minutes

Cook Time: 20 minutes

Serving Size: 1 toast
(makes 2 servings)

(Per Toast):

Calories: 210

Carbs: 30g

Sugar: 6g

Protein: 4g

Fat: 9g

1 medium sweet potato

1 avocado, mashed

1/2 teaspoon ground cinnamon

1/4 teaspoon salt

1 tablespoon olive oil

Toppings: sliced tomatoes, arugula, or microgreens

Red pepper flakes or sesame seeds for garnish

Preheat the oven to 400 °F (200 °C). Cut the sweet potato into 1/4-inch thick slices (lengthwise).

Place the sweet potato slices on a baking sheet lined with parchment paper. Drizzle olive oil and season with salt. Roast for 20 minutes, turning halfway through, until soft and faintly crusty.

While the sweet potato roasts, mash the avocado in a small bowl. If desired, mix in ground cinnamon and season with salt to taste.

Once the sweet potato slices are done, take them out of the oven. Spread the mashed avocado on top of each slice.

If preferred, top with sliced tomatoes, arugula, or microgreens. Before serving, garnish with sesame seeds or red pepper flakes.

Potato and Egg Muffins

Prep Time: 10 minutes

Cook Time: 25 minutes

Serving Size: 1 muffin (makes 6 servings)

(Per Muffin):

Calories: 150

Carbs: 15g

Sugar: 1g

Protein: 6g

Fat: 8g

2 medium potatoes, grated (about 2 cups)

4 large eggs

1/2 cup diced bell pepper (any color)

1/2 cup chopped spinach (fresh or frozen)

1/4 cup grated cheese (such as cheddar or feta)

1 teaspoon garlic powder

1/2 teaspoon salt

1/4 teaspoon black pepper

Olive oil spray or muffin liners

Set the oven to 375°F (190°C). Lightly coat a muffin tray with olive oil or line it with muffin liners.

In a large mixing dish, add shredded potatoes, diced bell pepper, spinach, garlic powder, salt, and pepper. Mix thoroughly.

In a separate dish, whisk the eggs before pouring them into the potato mixture. Stir until everything is well incorporated. If using cheese, fold it in at this point.

Spoon the potato and egg mixture equally into the muffin cups, filling them approximately three-quarters full.

Bake in a preheated oven for 20-25 minutes, or until the muffins are firm and gently brown on top.

Allow the muffins to cool for a few minutes before removing from the pan. Serve warm or room temperature.

Quick Chia Pudding

Prep Time: 5 minutes

Cook Time: 0 minutes (plus chilling time)

Serving Size: 1 cup (makes 2 servings)

(Per Cup):

Calories: 240

Carbs: 34g

Sugar: 10g

Protein: 6g

Fat: 10g

1/2 cup chia seeds

2 cups unsweetened almond milk

2 tablespoons maple syrup or honey

1 teaspoon vanilla extract

fresh fruits (like berries or banana), nuts, coconut flakes, or granola (optional)

In a medium bowl, mix together chia seeds, almond milk, maple syrup or honey (if using), and vanilla essence until completely incorporated.

Cover the bowl and chill for at least 4 hours, or overnight, until the mixture reaches a pudding-like consistency.

After chilling, give the chia pudding a thorough toss. If it's too thick, add a bit more almond milk until you have the right consistency.

Divide the pudding into two dishes or jars, then top with your favorite fresh fruits, nuts, coconut flakes, or granola..

Savory Oatmeal Bowl

Prep Time: 5 minutes

Cook Time: 10 minutes

Serving Size: 1 bowl (makes 2 servings)

(Per Bowl):

Calories: 310

Carbs: 40g

Sugar: 4g

Protein: 12g

Fat: 12g

- 1 cup rolled oats
- 2 cups water or low-sodium vegetable broth
- 1/2 cup diced tomatoes (fresh or canned)
- 1/2 cup chopped spinach or kale
- 1/4 cup grated Parmesan cheese (optional)
- 1 tablespoon olive oil
- 1/2 teaspoon garlic powder
- 1/4 teaspoon salt
- 1/4 teaspoon black pepper
- 2 large eggs
- Fresh herbs (like basil or parsley) for garnish

In a medium saucepan, heat the water or vegetable broth until it boils. Mix in the rolled oats, garlic powder, salt, and pepper. Reduce the heat to medium and simmer for 5-7 minutes, stirring regularly, until the oats become creamy and soft.

In the last minute of simmering, toss in the diced tomatoes and chopped spinach or kale until wilted. Remove from heat.

In a separate pan, warm the olive oil over medium heat. Crack the eggs into the skillet and cook according to your desire.

Divide the flavorful oatmeal into two dishes. Top each bowl with a cooked egg (if using), then sprinkle with grated Parmesan cheese and fresh herbs.

Enjoy your oatmeal warm, drizzling with more olive oil as needed..

Roasted Potato Tacos

Prep Time: 10 minutes

Cook Time: 25 minutes

Serving Size: 2 tacos (makes 4 servings)

(Per Taco):

Calories: 220

Carbs: 30g

Sugar: 2g

Protein: 6g

Fat: 8g

2 medium sweet potatoes, diced (about 2 cups)

1 tablespoon olive oil

1 teaspoon paprika

1/2 teaspoon garlic powder

1/2 teaspoon cumin

1/4 teaspoon salt

1/4 teaspoon black pepper

8 small corn tortillas

4 large eggs

1/2 avocado, sliced

Fresh cilantro, chopped

Salsa or hot sauce (for serving,)

Set your oven to 425°F (220°C). Line a baking sheet with parchment paper.

In a large bowl, combine the diced sweet potatoes, olive oil, paprika, garlic powder, cumin, salt, and black pepper. Spread the seasoned potatoes equally on the prepared baking sheet. Roast for 20-25 minutes, or until soft and mildly crispy, tossing halfway through.

While the potatoes are roasting, prepare the eggs as desired (scrambled, fried, or poached).

In a pan over medium heat, cook the corn tortillas for approximately 30 seconds on each side until malleable.

Once the potatoes are cooked, take them out of the oven. Divide the roasted sweet potatoes and fried eggs between the heated tortillas. Garnish with sliced avocado and chopped cilantro.

If preferred, drizzle with salsa or spicy sauce and eat your morning tacos while still warm..

Rice Bowl

Prep Time: 10 minutes

Cook Time: 20 minutes

Serving Size: 1 bowl (makes 2 servings)

(Per Bowl):

Calories: 360

Carbs: 55g

Sugar: 3g

Protein: 12g

Fat: 12g

- 1 cup brown rice (or quinoa)
- 2 cups water or low-sodium vegetable broth
- 1 cup cooked chickpeas (canned or homemade)
- 1 cup steamed broccoli florets
- 1/2 cup diced carrots
- 1/2 avocado, sliced
- 1 tablespoon olive oil
- 1 teaspoon turmeric powder
- 1 teaspoon garlic powder
- 1/2 teaspoon salt
- 1/4 teaspoon black pepper
- Fresh lemon juice (for drizzling)
- Fresh herbs (like parsley or cilantro) for garnish

In a medium saucepan, heat the water or vegetable broth until it boils. Combine the brown rice, turmeric powder, garlic powder, salt, and black pepper. Reduce the heat to low, cover, and cook for about 40-45 minutes, or until the rice is cooked and the liquid has been absorbed. (If using quinoa, follow the cooking time specified on the box).

While the rice cooks, steam the broccoli florets and sliced carrots until soft (5-7 minutes).

When the rice is done, fluff it with a fork and divide it into two bowls. Top each bowl with cooked chickpeas, steamed broccoli, chopped carrots, and sliced avocado.

Drizzle the bowls with olive oil and fresh lemon juice. Garnish with fresh herbs if desired.

Warm your Anti-Inflammatory Rice Bowl for a nutritious lunch or supper.

Quick Apple-Carrot Oats

Prep Time: 5 minutes

Cook Time: 5 minutes

Serving Size: 1 bowl (makes 2 servings)

(Per Bowl):

Calories: 240

Carbs: 42g

Sugar: 10g

Protein: 6g

Fat: 4g

1 cup rolled oats

2 cups water or unsweetened almond milk

1 medium apple, grated (about 1 cup)

1 medium carrot, grated (about 1 cup)

1 teaspoon cinnamon

1 tablespoon maple syrup or honey

1/4 cup raisins or chopped nuts

A pinch of salt

Fresh apple slices for garnish

In a medium saucepan, heat the water or almond milk until it boils. Mix in the rolled oats, grated apple, carrot, cinnamon, and salt.

Lower the heat to low and simmer for 5 minutes, stirring regularly, until the oats are creamy and the mixture thickens.

If preferred, add maple syrup or honey in the final minute of cooking.

Divide the oats into two dishes. If desired, top with raisins or chopped almonds and garnish with fresh apple slices..

Sheet Pan Breakfast

Prep Time: 10 minutes

Cook Time: 25 minutes

Serving Size: 1/2 pan (makes 4 servings)

(Per Serving):

Calories: 300

Carbs: 30g

Sugar: 5g

Protein: 12g

Fat: 15g

4 medium sweet potatoes, diced (about 4 cups)

1 cup cherry tomatoes, halved

1 cup broccoli florets

1 bell pepper, diced

8 large eggs

2 tablespoons olive oil

1 teaspoon garlic powder

1 teaspoon paprika

1/2 teaspoon salt

1/4 teaspoon black pepper

Fresh herbs (like parsley or cilantro) for garnish

Preheat the oven to 400 degrees Fahrenheit (200 degrees Celsius). Line a large sheet pan with parchment paper.

In a large mixing bowl, combine the diced sweet potatoes, cherry tomatoes, broccoli florets, and bell pepper with the olive oil, garlic powder, paprika, salt, and black pepper.

Distribute the seasoned veggies equally on the prepared sheet pan.

Cook the veggies in a preheated oven for 20 minutes.

Take out the pan from the oven. Make eight tiny wells in the roasted veggies and place one egg in each. Return the pan to the oven and bake for another 5-7 minutes, or until the eggs are cooked to your preference.

Remove from the oven, sprinkle with fresh herbs if preferred, and serve warm..

SALADS, WRAPS AND LIGHT MEALS

Mediterranean Quinoa Bowl

Prep Time: 10 minutes

Cook Time: 15 minutes

Serving Size: 1 bowl (makes 2 servings)

1 cup quinoa, rinsed

2 cups water or low-sodium vegetable broth

1 cup cherry tomatoes, halved

1 cup cucumber, diced

1/2 cup Kalamata olives, pitted and halved

1/4 cup red onion, finely chopped

1/2 cup feta cheese, crumbled (optional)

2 tablespoons olive oil

1 tablespoon lemon juice

1 teaspoon dried oregano

Salt and pepper to taste

Fresh parsley or basil for garnish

(Per Bowl):

Calories: 320

Carbs: 36g

Sugar: 3g

Protein: 10g

Fat: 15g

Heat water or vegetable broth in a medium pot until it boils. Add the rinsed quinoa, lower heat to low, cover, and cook for approximately 15 minutes, or until the quinoa is fluffy and the liquid has been absorbed. Remove from heat, cover, and allow to sit for 5 minutes before fluffing with a fork.

In a large bowl, mix the cherry tomatoes, cucumber, Kalamata olives, red onion, and feta cheese (if using).

In a small bowl, combine the olive oil, lemon juice, dried oregano, salt, and pepper. Toss the vegetables with the dressing until well combined.

Place the cooked quinoa in two bowls and top with the Mediterranean vegetable combination.

Garnish with fresh parsley or basil. Serve.

Wild Salmon & Berry Salad

Prep Time: 10 minutes

Cook Time: 15 minutes

Serving Size: 1 bowl (makes 2 servings)

(Per Bowl):

Calories: 350

Carbohydrates: 18g

Sugar: 5g

Protein: 30g

Fat: 20g

- 2 (4-ounce) wild salmon filets
- 1 tablespoon olive oil
- Salt and pepper to taste
- 4 cups mixed greens (spinach, arugula, or kale)
- 1 cup mixed berries
- 1/2 cup cucumber, sliced
- 1/4 cup red onion, thinly sliced
- 1/4 cup walnuts or pecans, chopped (optional)
- 2 tablespoons balsamic vinaigrette or lemon juice for dressing

Preheat the oven to 400 °F (200 °C). Arrange the salmon filets on a baking pan lined with parchment paper. Drizzle with olive oil, then season with salt and pepper. Bake for 12-15 minutes, or until the salmon is well cooked and readily flaked with a fork.

While the salmon cooks, combine the mixed greens, mixed berries, sliced cucumber, and red onion in a large bowl. Toss lightly to combine.

Sprinkle chopped walnuts or pecans over the salad.

After the salmon is cooked, let it rest for a minute before flaking it into big pieces. Divide the salad into two dishes and top with the flakes salmon.

Drizzle balsamic vinaigrette or lemon juice on top before serving..

Turmeric Roasted Cauliflower Salad

Prep Time: 10 minutes

Cook Time: 25 minutes

Serving Size: 1 bowl (makes 4 servings)

(Per Serving):

Calories: 180

Carbs: 16g

Sugar: 3g

Protein: 5g

Fat: 12g

- 1 medium head of cauliflower, cut into florets (about 4 cups)
- 2 tablespoons olive oil
- 1 teaspoon turmeric powder
- 1 teaspoon cumin
- 1/2 teaspoon garlic powder
- 1/2 teaspoon salt
- 1/4 teaspoon black pepper
- 4 cups mixed greens (spinach, arugula, or kale)
- 1/2 cup cherry tomatoes, halved
- 1/4 cup red onion, thinly sliced
- 1/4 cup feta cheese (optional, omit for dairy-free)
- 1/4 cup chopped fresh parsley or cilantro
- Lemon wedges

Set your oven to 425°F (220°C) and prepare a baking sheet with parchment paper.

In a large mixing bowl, combine the cauliflower florets, olive oil, turmeric powder, cumin, garlic powder, salt, and black pepper.

Arrange the seasoned cauliflower in a single layer on the prepared baking sheet. Roast for 25-30 minutes, or until golden brown and delicious. Flip halfway through.

In a large mixing bowl, add the mixed greens, roasted cauliflower, cherry tomatoes, red onion, feta cheese (if desired), and chopped parsley or cilantro.

Drizzle with more olive oil and lemon juice, if preferred. Toss lightly to mix, then serve

Greek Kale Bowl

Prep Time: 10 minutes

Cook Time: 15 minutes

Serving Size: 1 bowl (makes 2 servings)

(Per Bowl):

Calories: 320

Carbs: 30g

Sugar: 3g

Protein: 10g

Fat: 18g

- 4 cups kale, chopped
- 1 cup cooked quinoa (or brown rice)
- 1 cup cherry tomatoes, halved
- 1/2 cucumber, diced
- 1/2 cup Kalamata olives, pitted and sliced
- 1/2 cup crumbled feta cheese (omit for dairy-free)
- 1/4 cup red onion, thinly sliced
- 1 tablespoon olive oil
- 1 tablespoon red wine vinegar
- 1 teaspoon dried oregano
- Salt and pepper, to taste
- Fresh lemon wedges (for serving)

If the quinoa has not previously been cooked, follow the package directions. Set aside.

In a large bowl, combine the chopped kale, olive oil, and a teaspoon of salt. Massage the kale for 1-2 minutes until it softens and lowers in volume.

Mix the cooked quinoa, cherry tomatoes, cucumber, olives, feta cheese (if using), and red onion into the massaged kale.

In a small bowl, combine the red wine vinegar, dried oregano, salt, and pepper. Drizzle the dressing over the kale mixture and toss until well mixed.

Separate the Greek Kale Power Bowl onto two plates or bowls. Serve with fresh lemon wedges on the side for an added blast of flavor..

Collard Green Turkey Wrap

Prep Time: 10 minutes

Cook Time: 0 minutes

Serving Size: 1 wrap (makes 4 servings)

(Per Wrap):

Calories: 180

Carbs: 14g

Sugar: 2g

Protein: 20g

Fat: 7g

- 4 large collard green leaves
- 8 ounces sliced turkey breast (deli meat or cooked turkey)
- 1/2 cup hummus or avocado spread
- 1/2 cup grated carrots
- 1/2 cup cucumber, thinly sliced
- 1/2 cup bell pepper, thinly sliced
- 1/4 cup red onion, thinly sliced
- Salt and pepper to taste
- Fresh herbs (like cilantro or parsley) for garnish

Rinse the collard green leaves completely, then clip the thick stem at the bottom. To make the leaves more malleable, blanch them in boiling water for 30 seconds before transferring them to an ice bath to chill, or use them raw if tender enough.

Place a collard green leaf flat on a clean surface. Spread 2 tablespoons of hummus or avocado equally over each leaf.

Place 2 ounces of sliced turkey on top of the spread. Add some grated carrots, cucumber slices, bell pepper slices, and red onion.

Add salt and pepper to taste.

Beginning at one end, firmly wrap the collard green leaf snugly around the contents. Tuck in the sides as you roll to keep the contents within.

Repeat with the remaining leaves and filling. Cut each wrap in half and serve, topped with fresh herbs as desired.

Mediterranean Hummus Wrap

Prep Time: 10 minutes

Cook Time: 0 minutes

Serving Size: 1 wrap (makes 2 servings)

(Per Wrap):

Calories: 280

Carbs: 40g

Sugar: 3g

Protein: 10g

Fat: 10g

- 2 large whole grain or gluten-free tortillas
- 1 cup hummus (store-bought or homemade)
- 1 cup mixed salad greens (spinach, arugula, or romaine)
- 1/2 cup diced cucumber
- 1/2 cup diced tomatoes
- 1/4 cup sliced red onion
- 1/4 cup feta cheese
- 1/4 cup kalamata olives, pitted and sliced
- 1 tablespoon olive oil
- 1 tablespoon lemon juice
- Salt and pepper to taste
- Fresh herbs (like parsley or dill) for garnish

In a mixing bowl, add the chopped cucumber, tomatoes, red onion, kalamata olives, olive oil, lemon juice, salt, and pepper. Toss to blend.

Place the tortillas flat on a clean surface. Spread 1/2 cup hummus evenly on each tortilla.

Layer the mixed salad greens on top of the hummus, followed by the cucumber-tomato combination. Sprinkle with feta cheese and fresh herbs, if desired.

Roll the tortilla firmly, tucking in the edges as you go, to form a wrap.

Cut the wraps in half and serve right away, or wrap in foil for an on-the-go dinner..

Asian-Style Lettuce Wraps

Prep Time: 15 minutes

Cook Time: 10 minutes

Serving Size: 2 wraps (makes 4 servings)

(Per Wrap):

Calories: 160

Carbs: 8g

Sugar: 2g

Protein: 20g

Fat: 7g

- 1 pound ground turkey or chicken
- 1 tablespoon sesame oil
- 2 cloves garlic, minced
- 1-inch piece fresh ginger, minced
- 1/2 cup diced bell pepper
- 1/2 cup grated carrots
- 1/2 cup water chestnuts, diced
- 1/4 cup low-sodium soy sauce or tamari
- 1 tablespoon rice vinegar
- 1 tablespoon honey or maple syrup
- 1/2 teaspoon red pepper flakes
- 8 large lettuce leaves (like butter or romaine)
- Fresh cilantro or green onions for garnish

In a large pan, heat the sesame oil over medium heat. Cook the ground turkey or chicken until browned and cooked thoroughly, approximately 5-7 minutes.

Stir in the minced garlic and ginger and simmer for another 1-2 minutes, or until fragrant.

Combine the diced bell pepper, shredded carrots, and water chestnuts. Cook for another 3-4 minutes, stirring regularly.

In a small mixing dish, combine soy sauce, rice vinegar, honey or maple syrup, and red pepper flakes (if used). Pour the sauce over the meat and veggies and toss to mix. Cook for another 2-3 minutes, until well heated.

Spoon the mixture into the middle of each lettuce leaf and fold them into tacos.

If preferred, garnish with fresh cilantro or green onions, then enjoy your Asian-Style Lettuce Wraps.

Ginger-Turmeric Salmon Bowl

Prep Time: 10 minutes

Cook Time: 15 minutes

Serving Size: 1 bowl (makes 2 servings)

(Per Bowl):

Calories: 450

Carbs: 30g

Sugar: 2g

Protein: 32g

Fat: 24g

2 salmon filets (about 6 oz each)

1 tablespoon olive oil

1 teaspoon ground turmeric

1 teaspoon ground ginger (or 1 tablespoon fresh ginger, grated)

1/2 teaspoon garlic powder

1/4 teaspoon salt

1/4 teaspoon black pepper

1 cup cooked quinoa (or brown rice)

1 cup steamed broccoli florets

1/2 cup diced cucumber

1/2 avocado, sliced

Fresh lemon wedges (for serving)

Fresh cilantro for garnish

Preheat the oven to 400 degrees Fahrenheit (200 degrees Celsius).

In a small bowl, combine the olive oil, turmeric, ginger, garlic powder, salt, and black pepper. Rub the mixture on both sides of the salmon filets.

Arrange the salmon filets on a baking sheet lined with parchment paper. Bake for 12-15 minutes, or until the salmon is well cooked and readily flaked with a fork.

While the salmon bakes, make the quinoa (or rice) and steam the broccoli, if not already done. Divide the cooked quinoa into two bowls, then top with steamed broccoli, chopped cucumber, and sliced avocado.

When the salmon is cooked, lay one filet in each dish.

Finish with fresh cilantro and lemon wedges. Squeeze lemon juice over the dish to add flavor.

Mediterranean Chickpea Bowl

Prep Time: 10 minutes

Cook Time: 10 minutes

Serving Size: 1 bowl (makes 2 servings)

(Per Bowl):

Calories: 360

Carbs: 48g

Sugar: 6g

Protein: 12g

Fat: 14g

- 1 cup cooked chickpeas (canned or homemade, drained and rinsed)
- 1 cup cooked quinoa or brown rice
- 1 cup diced cucumber
- 1 cup cherry tomatoes, halved
- 1/2 cup red onion, finely chopped
- 1/4 cup Kalamata olives, sliced
- 1/4 cup feta cheese (optional)
- 2 tablespoons olive oil
- 1 tablespoon lemon juice
- 1 teaspoon dried oregano
- Salt and pepper to taste
- Fresh parsley for garnish

In a bowl, mix cooked quinoa or brown rice to form the basis of your Mediterranean bowl.

In a separate dish, mix together the chickpeas, chopped cucumber, cherry tomatoes, red onion, and Kalamata olives. If using, include feta cheese into the mixture.

In a small bowl, combine the olive oil, lemon juice, dried oregano, salt, and pepper. Toss together the chickpea mixture and dressing.

Spoon the chickpea salad over the quinoa or brown rice foundation.

If preferred, add fresh parsley to your Mediterranean Chickpea Bowl.

Sweet Potato & Black Bean Buddha Bowl

Prep Time: 10 minutes

Cook Time: 25 minutes

Serving Size: 1 bowl (makes 2 servings)

(Per Bowl):

Calories: 400

Carbs: 60g

Sugar: 6g

Protein: 14g

Fat: 14g

- 1 medium sweet potato, diced (about 1 cup)
- 1 tablespoon olive oil
- 1/2 teaspoon paprika
- 1/2 teaspoon garlic powder
- 1/4 teaspoon salt
- 1/4 teaspoon black pepper
- 1 can (15 oz) black beans, rinsed and drained
- 2 cups cooked quinoa or brown rice
- 1 cup chopped kale or spinach
- 1/2 avocado, sliced
- Fresh cilantro, chopped
- Lime wedges (for serving)

Set your oven to 425°F (220°C) and prepare a baking sheet with parchment paper.

In a bowl, combine the diced sweet potatoes, olive oil, paprika, garlic powder, salt, and black pepper. Spread them out equally on the prepared baking sheet. Roast for 20-25 minutes, or until soft and mildly crispy, tossing halfway through.

While the sweet potatoes roast, carefully sauté the chopped kale or spinach in a small pan over medium heat until wilted (3-4 minutes).

Divide the cooked quinoa or brown rice into two dishes. Top each dish with roasted sweet potatoes, black beans, sautéed greens, and sliced avocado.

Add fresh cilantro and lime wedges on the side.

Rainbow Poke Bowl

Prep Time: 15 minutes

Cook Time: 15 minutes (for rice)

Serving Size: 1 bowl (makes 2 servings)

(Per Bowl):

Calories: 380

Carbs: 55g

Sugar: 4g

Protein: 15g

Fat: 12g

- 1 cup sushi rice (or brown rice)
- 1 1/2 cups water
- 1 tablespoon rice vinegar
- 1 tablespoon sesame oil
- 1 teaspoon soy sauce (or tamari for gluten-free)
- 1/2 teaspoon salt
- 1 cup diced cucumber
- 1 cup shredded carrots
- 1 cup sliced radishes
- 1 cup diced avocado
- 1 cup cubed tofu (or cooked shrimp for non-vegetarian option)
- 1/4 cup edamame (shelled)
- 1 tablespoon sesame seeds (for garnish)
- Fresh cilantro or green onions for garnish

In a medium saucepan, mix the sushi rice and water. Bring to a boil, then lower to a low heat, cover, and simmer for 15 minutes, or until the rice is cooked and the water has been absorbed. Remove from the heat and let it settle for 5 minutes, covered.

In a small dish, combine rice vinegar, sesame oil, soy sauce, and salt.

Using a fork, fluff the cooked rice and sprinkle in the dressing. Stir to mix and let cool slightly.

Separate the seasoned rice into two bowls. Place the chopped cucumber, shredded carrots, sliced radishes, diced avocado, cubed tofu (or shrimp), and edamame in portions on top of the rice.

Top with sesame seeds and, if preferred, fresh cilantro or green onions. Serve.

Lentil & Roasted Vegetable Bowl

Prep Time: 15 minutes

Cook Time: 30 minutes

Serving Size: 1 bowl (makes 4 servings)

(Per Bowl):

Calories: 320

Carbs: 55g

Sugar: 5g

Protein: 15g

Fat: 8g

- 1 cup green or brown lentils, rinsed
- 3 cups water or low-sodium vegetable broth
- 2 cups mixed vegetables (like bell peppers, zucchini, and carrots), diced
- 1 tablespoon olive oil
- 1 teaspoon garlic powder
- 1 teaspoon smoked paprika
- 1/2 teaspoon salt
- 1/4 teaspoon black pepper
- 1/2 teaspoon dried thyme or rosemary
- Fresh parsley or cilantro for garnish

Set your oven to 425°F (220°C) and prepare a baking sheet with parchment paper.

In a bowl, combine the chopped mixed vegetables, olive oil, and garlic powder, smoked paprika, salt, black pepper, and dried thyme. Spread the veggies equally on the prepared baking sheet. Roast for 20-25 minutes, or until soft and faintly caramelized, stirring halfway through.

In a medium saucepan, heat the water or vegetable broth to a boil while the veggies roast. Combine the washed lentils with a sprinkle of salt. Reduce the heat to low, cover, and cook for about 20-25 minutes, or until the lentils are soft but not mushy.

Once the lentils and veggies have been cooked, divide them into four bowls. Top each dish with the roasted veggies.

If preferred, garnish with fresh parsley or cilantro and enjoy your healthful **Lentil & Roasted Vegetable Bowl** while still warm..

Greek Shrimp Salad

Prep Time: 10 minutes

Cook Time: 5 minutes

Serving Size: 1 bowl (makes 2 servings)

(Per Bowl):

Calories: 320

Carbs: 12g

Sugar: 3g

Protein: 28g

Fat: 20g

- 1 pound large shrimp, peeled and deveined
- 2 tablespoons olive oil
- 1 teaspoon dried oregano
- 1/2 teaspoon garlic powder
- Salt and pepper to taste
- 4 cups mixed salad greens (such as spinach, arugula, and romaine)
- 1 cup cherry tomatoes, halved
- 1 cucumber, diced
- 1/4 red onion, thinly sliced
- 1/2 cup Kalamata olives, pitted and halved
- 1/2 cup feta cheese, crumbled (optional)
- Fresh lemon juice for dressing

In a medium mixing bowl, combine the shrimp, olive oil, oregano, garlic powder, salt, and pepper.

Place a skillet over medium-high heat. Cook the seasoned shrimp for 2-3 minutes on each side, or until pink and opaque. Remove from heat.

In a large bowl, combine the mixed salad greens, cherry tomatoes, cucumber, red onion, and Kalamata olives. Toss to mix.

Top the salad with cooked shrimp and, if desired, sprinkle with feta cheese.

Drizzle the salad with fresh lemon juice before serving..

Roasted Vegetable & Quinoa Bowl

Prep Time: 10 minutes

Cook Time: 30 minutes

Serving Size: 1 bowl (makes 2 servings)

(Per Bowl):

Calories: 320

Carbs: 45g

Sugar: 4g

Protein: 10g

Fat: 12g

1 cup quinoa

2 cups water or low-sodium vegetable broth

1 red bell pepper, diced

1 zucchini, diced

1 cup broccoli florets

1 carrot, sliced

2 tablespoons olive oil

1 teaspoon garlic powder

1 teaspoon paprika

1/2 teaspoon salt

1/4 teaspoon black pepper

1/4 cup hummus

Fresh lemon juice (for drizzling)

Fresh herbs (like parsley or cilantro) for garnish

Set your oven to 425°F (220°C). Line a baking sheet with parchment paper.

In a medium saucepan, heat the water or vegetable broth until it boils. Add the quinoa, decrease the heat to low, cover, and cook for 15 minutes, or until the quinoa is tender and fluffy. Remove from the heat and put aside.

In a large mixing bowl, combine the chopped bell pepper, zucchini, broccoli, and carrot with olive oil, garlic powder, paprika, salt, and black pepper. Spread the veggies equally on the prepared baking sheet. Roast for 20-25 minutes, or until soft and faintly caramelized, stirring halfway through.

Divide the cooked quinoa into two dishes. Top each dish with roasted veggies and a dab of hummus, if desired.

Drizzle with lemon juice and garnish with fresh herbs, if preferred..

Wild Rice & Cranberry Salad

Prep Time: 10 minutes

Cook Time: 40 minutes

Serving Size: 1 cup (makes 4 servings)

(Per Serving):

Calories: 240

Carbs: 32g

Sugar: 6g

Protein: 6g

Fat: 10g

- 1 cup wild rice
- 3 cups water or low-sodium vegetable broth
- 1/2 cup dried cranberries
- 1/2 cup diced celery
- 1/2 cup diced red bell pepper
- 1/4 cup chopped fresh parsley
- 1/4 cup chopped walnuts or pecans (optional)
- 1/4 cup olive oil
- 2 tablespoons apple cider vinegar
- 1 tablespoon Dijon mustard
- 1 teaspoon maple syrup (optional)
- Salt and pepper to taste

Rinse it with cool water. In a medium saucepan, mix the wild rice, water, or vegetable broth. Bring to a boil, then decrease heat to low, cover, and cook for 40-45 minutes, or until rice is soft and liquid has been absorbed. Drain any surplus liquid as needed.

After cooking, remove it from the heat and allow it to cool to room temperature.

In a small mixing bowl, combine olive oil, apple cider vinegar, Dijon mustard, maple syrup (if using), salt, and pepper.

In a large mixing dish, add cooled wild rice, dried cranberries, diced celery, diced red bell pepper, chopped parsley, and nuts (if using). Pour the dressing over the salad and toss to mix.

Add more salt and pepper to taste. Serve or chill for 30 minutes to let the flavors combine..

Mediterranean Tuna Salad

Prep Time: 10 minutes

Cook Time: 0 minutes

Serving Size: 1 cup (makes 2 servings)

(Per Serving):

Calories: 260

Carbs: 10g

Sugar: 2g

Protein: 30g

Fat: 12g

- 1 can (5 oz) tuna in olive oil or water, drained
- 1/2 cup cherry tomatoes, halved
- 1/2 cucumber, diced
- 1/4 cup red onion, finely chopped
- 1/4 cup Kalamata olives, pitted and sliced
- 1/4 cup bell pepper, diced (any color)
- 2 tablespoons fresh parsley, chopped
- 2 tablespoons olive oil
- 1 tablespoon red wine vinegar or lemon juice
- 1/2 teaspoon dried oregano
- Salt and pepper to taste

In a large mixing bowl, add drained tuna, cherry tomatoes, cucumber, red onion, olives, bell pepper, and parsley.

In a small bowl, combine the olive oil, red wine vinegar (or lemon juice), dried oregano, salt, and pepper.

Pour the dressing over the tuna mixture and gently toss until well incorporated.

Divide the Mediterranean tuna salad between two dishes, or serve over greens or in pita bread..

Grilled Chicken & Avocado Lettuce Cups

Prep Time: 10 minutes

Cook Time: 10 minutes

Serving Size: 2 cups (makes 4 servings)

(Per Cup):

Calories: 210

Carbs: 8g

Sugar: 1g

Protein: 22g

Fat: 11g

2 large chicken breasts (about 1 pound)

1 tablespoon olive oil

1 teaspoon garlic powder

1 teaspoon paprika

1/2 teaspoon salt

1/4 teaspoon black pepper

1 avocado, diced

1 cup cherry tomatoes, halved

1/4 cup red onion, finely chopped

1 tablespoon fresh lime juice

8 large romaine or butter lettuce leaves

In a dish, mix together olive oil, garlic powder, paprika, salt, and black pepper. Add the chicken breasts and coat evenly with the marinade. Allow it to settle for around 5-10 minutes.

Preheat the grill or grill pan to medium-high heat. Grill the chicken breasts for 5-7 minutes each side, or until thoroughly cooked (internal temperature should be 165°F/74°C). Remove off the grill and let it rest for a few minutes before slicing.

In a mixing dish, add chopped avocado, cherry tomatoes, red onion, and lime juice. Gently mix until combined.

Place one lettuce leaf on a platter. Top with sliced grilled chicken and avocado mixture. Repeat for the remaining leaves..

Beet & Goat Cheese Salad

Prep Time: 15 minutes

Cook Time: 30 minutes (if roasting beets)

Serving Size: 1 salad (makes 2 servings)

(Per Salad):

Calories: 290

Carbs: 22g

Sugar: 6g

Protein: 8g

Fat: 20g

- 2 medium beets, roasted and sliced (or 1 cup pre-cooked beets)
- 4 cups mixed greens (like arugula, spinach, or kale)
- 1/4 cup crumbled goat cheese
- 1/4 cup walnuts, toasted
- 1/2 cup sliced cucumbers
- 1/4 cup red onion, thinly sliced
- 2 tablespoons balsamic vinegar
- 1 tablespoon olive oil
- Salt and pepper to taste

Preheat the oven to 400 °F (200 °C). Wrap the beets in foil and put them on a baking pan. Roast for 30-40 minutes, or until fork-tender. Allow to cool, then peel and slice.

In a large bowl, add the mixed greens, sliced beets, cucumbers, red onion, and walnuts.

In a small bowl, combine the balsamic vinegar, olive oil, salt, and pepper to taste.

Drizzle the dressing over the salad and gently toss to mix. Top with crumbled goat cheese.

Place the salad on two plates and serve as a light lunch or side dish..

Miso Glazed Tofu Bowl

Prep Time: 15 minutes

Cook Time: 25 minutes

Serving Size: 1 bowl (makes 2 servings)

(Per Bowl):

Calories: 400

Carbs: 52g

Sugar: 6g

Protein: 18g

Fat: 14g

14 oz (400g) firm tofu, drained and pressed

2 tablespoons miso paste (white or yellow)

2 tablespoons soy sauce (or tamari for gluten-free)

1 tablespoon maple syrup or honey

1 tablespoon rice vinegar

1 tablespoon sesame oil

1 cup cooked brown rice or quinoa

1 cup steamed broccoli florets

1/2 cup shredded carrots

1/4 cup green onions, sliced

Sesame seeds (for garnish)

Fresh cilantro or parsley

Preheat the oven to 400 degrees Fahrenheit (200 degrees Celsius). Line a baking sheet with parchment paper.

Cut the squeezed tofu into cubes. In a medium mixing bowl, combine the miso paste, soy sauce, maple syrup, rice vinegar, and sesame oil until smooth. Add the tofu cubes and gently toss to coat with the marinade.

Place the marinated tofu cubes on the prepared baking sheet in a single layer. Bake for 20-25 minutes, turning halfway through, until the tofu becomes golden and somewhat crispy.

While the tofu bakes, cook the brown rice or quinoa according to package directions, if not already done. Steam broccoli florets till tender.

Divide the cooked rice or quinoa into two dishes. Top each dish with roasted miso-glazed tofu, steamed broccoli, shredded carrots, and thinly sliced green onions.

Top with sesame seeds and fresh cilantro or parsley, if preferred. Serve your Miso Glazed Tofu Bowl warm.

VEGETARIAN AND VEGAN

Cauliflower-Walnut "Sausage"

Prep Time: 15 minutes

Cook Time: 20 minutes

Serving Size: 2 stuffed peppers (makes 4 servings)

(Per Stuffed Pepper):

Calories: 160

Carbs: 12g

Sugar: 3g

Protein: 5g

Fat: 12g

8 Peppadew peppers (or similar-sized sweet peppers)

1 cup cauliflower florets, finely chopped

1 cup walnuts, finely chopped

1/2 cup cooked quinoa (or brown rice)

2 cloves garlic, minced

1 teaspoon dried oregano

1 teaspoon smoked paprika

1/2 teaspoon salt

1/4 teaspoon black pepper

2 tablespoons nutritional yeast

2 tablespoons olive oil, divided

Set your oven to 375°F (190°C).

In a large skillet, warm 1 tablespoon olive oil over medium heat. Sauté the minced garlic for approximately a minute, until fragrant. Next, add the chopped cauliflower and walnuts. Cook for 5-7 minutes, until the cauliflower is soft.

In a mixing dish, combine sautéed cauliflower and walnuts with cooked quinoa, oregano, smoked paprika, salt, black pepper, and nutritional yeast (if using). Mix well to mix.

Carefully remove the tops of the Peppadew peppers and discard any seeds. Fill each pepper with the cauliflower-walnut mixture, gently pushing down to pack it in.

Transfer the stuffed peppers to a baking sheet and sprinkle with the remaining tablespoon of olive oil. Bake for 15-20 minutes, or until the peppers are soft and the mixture has warmed through.

Jackfruit and Mushroom Wellington

Prep Time: 20 minutes

Cook Time: 45 minutes

Serving Size: 1 slice (makes 6 servings)

(Per Slice):

Calories: 290

Carbs: 36g

Sugar: 3g

Protein: 6g

Fat: 14g

1 can young green jackfruit in brine or water (about 20 oz), drained and rinsed

1 cup diced mushrooms (such as cremini or button)

1 small onion, diced

2 cloves garlic, minced

1 cup fresh spinach, chopped

1 tablespoon soy sauce or tamari (for gluten-free)

1 teaspoon smoked paprika

1 teaspoon dried thyme

1/2 teaspoon salt

1/4 teaspoon black pepper

1 sheet puff pastry (thawed if frozen)

1 tablespoon olive oil

1 tablespoon flour (for dusting)

1 tablespoon plant-based milk (for egg wash)

Preheat the oven to 400 degrees Fahrenheit (200 degrees Celsius). Line a baking sheet with parchment paper.

In a large skillet, heat the olive oil over medium heat. Sauté diced onion and garlic until softened, approximately 3-4 minutes. Cook for another 5 minutes, until the mushrooms have released their moisture and become soft.

Shred the jackfruit with a fork or your hands, then add it to the skillet. Stir in the spinach, soy sauce, smoked paprika, thyme, salt, and black pepper. Cook for a further 5 minutes, until the spinach has wilted. Remove from the heat and allow the mixture to cool somewhat.

On a lightly floured board, lay out the puff pastry to a rectangle. Place the cooled jackfruit and mushroom mixture in the middle of the dough to make a log shape. Fold the dough over the filling and seal the edges by pushing them together. Place the Wellington on the prepared baking sheet, seam side down.

Brush the top of the Wellington with plant-based milk. Cut a few openings at the top to let steam escape. Bake in a preheated oven for 25-30 minutes, or until the crust becomes golden brown.

Allow the Wellington to cool for a few minutes before slicing. Serve warm, with your choice of side dish.

Turmeric Chickpea Flour Pizza

Prep Time: 10 minutes

Cook Time: 20 minutes

Serving Size: 1 pizza (makes 2 servings)

(Per Serving, 1/2 Pizza):

Calories: 250

Carbs: 32g

Sugar: 3g

Protein: 10g

Fat: 10g

- 1 cup chickpea flour (also known as besan)
- 1 cup water
- 1 teaspoon turmeric powder
- 1/2 teaspoon garlic powder
- 1/2 teaspoon salt
- 1/4 teaspoon black pepper
- 2 tablespoons olive oil (divided)
- 1 cup diced vegetables (such as bell peppers, onions, and zucchini)
- 1/2 cup tomato sauce
- 1/2 cup shredded dairy-free cheese
- Fresh basil or arugula for garnish

Set your oven to 425°F (220°C). Line a baking sheet with parchment paper or gently coat it with olive oil.

In a mixing basin, combine chickpea flour, water, turmeric powder, garlic powder, salt, and black pepper. Whisk until smooth.

Pour 1 tablespoon olive oil onto the baking sheet and distribute it evenly. Pour the chickpea flour batter onto the sheet and spread it evenly to make a circular pizza crust approximately 1/4 inch thick.

Place the baking sheet in a preheated oven for 15 minutes, or until the edges are brown and the crust is set.

Remove the crust from the oven and evenly sprinkle the tomato sauce on top. Sprinkle the diced veggies with dairy-free cheese, if desired.

Return the pizza to the oven and bake for an additional 5-7 minutes, or until the veggies are soft and the cheese has melted.

Remove from the oven, let cool slightly, and sprinkle with fresh basil or arugula, if preferred. Slice and serve your Turmeric Chickpea Flour Pizza warm!

Crispy Rice Paper "Bacon" Breakfast Stack

Prep Time: 10 minutes

Cook Time: 15 minutes

Serving Size: 1 stack (makes 2 servings)

(Per Stack):

Calories: 350

Carbs: 34g

Sugar: 2g

Protein: 14g

Fat: 16g

6 sheets rice paper

2 tablespoons soy sauce or tamari (for a gluten-free option)

1 teaspoon liquid smoke

1 tablespoon maple syrup

1 cup cooked quinoa

4 large eggs

1 cup spinach or kale, sautéed

1 avocado, sliced

Olive oil spray or a small amount of olive oil for cooking

Fresh herbs (like chives or parsley) for garnish

In a shallow plate, mix together the soy sauce, liquid smoke, and maple syrup. Dip each rice paper sheet into warm water for approximately 5 seconds, or until malleable. Place the rice paper flat and coat both sides with the soy sauce mixture. Place on a parchment-lined baking sheet.

Preheat the oven to 400 °F (200 °C). Bake the rice paper for 10-12 minutes, turning halfway, until crispy and golden.

While the rice paper bakes, prepare the quinoa according to package directions if it has not previously been cooked.

Place a pan over medium heat and liberally coat with olive oil. Crack the eggs into the pan and cook until desired doneness (fried, scrambled, or poached).

On a dish, arrange the cooked quinoa, sautéed spinach or kale, and eggs. Garnish with crispy rice paper "bacon" and sliced avocado.

Garnish with fresh herbs if preferred and eat your crispy breakfast stack warm.

Zucchini Rollatini with Macadamia "Ricotta"

Prep Time: 15 minutes

Cook Time: 25 minutes

Serving Size: 2 rolls (makes 4 servings)

(Per Roll):

Calories: 180

Carbs: 9g

Sugar: 3g

Protein: 5g

Fat: 15g

2 large zucchinis

1 cup macadamia nuts, soaked in water for 2 hours and drained

1/4 cup nutritional yeast

1 tablespoon lemon juice

1 teaspoon garlic powder

1/2 teaspoon salt

1/4 teaspoon black pepper

1 cup marinara sauce (low-sodium)

Fresh basil leaves, for garnish

Set your oven to 375°F (190°C). Lightly coat a baking dish with olive oil or cooking spray.

Slice the zucchini lengthwise into thin strips (approximately 1/8 inch thick) using a mandolin or sharp knife. You should receive around 12 strips. To remove moisture, lightly salt the strips and allow them to rest for approximately 10 minutes. Pat dry with a paper towel.

Prepare the macadamia "ricotta"** In a food processor, mix together the soaked macadamia nuts, nutritional yeast, lemon juice, garlic powder, salt, and black pepper. Process until smooth and creamy. Season to taste.

Place a spoonful of macadamia "ricotta" on one end of each zucchini strip. Roll the strip around the filling, then set it seam side down in the baking dish. Repeat with each strip.

Pour the marinara sauce over the zucchini rollatini, being sure to evenly coat them.

Place in a preheated oven for 20-25 minutes, or until the zucchini is soft and the sauce bubbles.

Top with fresh basil leaves if wanted and serve warm..

Tandoori Cauliflower Steaks

Prep Time: 10 minutes

Cook Time: 25 minutes

Serving Size: 1 steak (makes 4 servings)

(Per Steak):

Calories: 150

Carbs: 10g

Sugar: 3g

Protein: 6g

Fat: 9g

- 1 large head of cauliflower
- 1 cup plain yogurt (dairy or dairy-free)
- 2 tablespoons tandoori masala
- 1 tablespoon olive oil
- 1 teaspoon garlic powder
- 1 teaspoon ginger powder
- 1/2 teaspoon salt
- 1/4 teaspoon black pepper
- Fresh cilantro, chopped
- Lemon wedges

Remove the cauliflower leaves and slice into 1-inch-thick steaks. You should get approximately 4-6 steaks from a single head.

In a medium mixing bowl, blend the yogurt, tandoori masala, olive oil, garlic powder, ginger powder, salt, and black pepper until thoroughly incorporated.

Apply the tandoori marinade thoroughly on both sides of each cauliflower steak. Allow the steaks to marinade for at least 15 minutes (up to 2 hours in the refrigerator for added flavor).

Set your oven to 425°F (220°C). Line a baking sheet with parchment paper.

Arrange the marinated cauliflower steaks on the prepared baking sheet. Bake for 20-25 minutes, turning halfway through, until tender and a little charred.

Remove from the oven and top with chopped cilantro. Serve lemon slices on the side..

BBQ Pulled Hearts of Palm Sliders

Prep Time: 15 minutes

Cook Time: 15 minutes

Serving Size: 2 sliders (makes 4 servings)

(Per Slider):

Calories: 180

Carbs: 30g

Sugar: 6g

Protein: 4g

Fat: 5g

2 cans (14 oz each) hearts of palm, drained and shredded

1 cup BBQ sauce (look for low-sugar options)

8 small whole-grain slider buns or lettuce leaves (for a low-carb option)

1/2 cup coleslaw (store-bought or homemade)

1 tablespoon olive oil

1 teaspoon smoked paprika

1/2 teaspoon garlic powder

1/4 teaspoon onion powder

Salt and pepper to taste

Fresh cilantro for garnish

Prepare the heart of palm In a medium dish, shred the drained hearts of palm with a fork until they look like pulled pork.

Cook the mixture in a skillet over medium heat with olive oil. Once heated, mix in the shredded hearts of palm, smoked paprika, garlic powder, onion powder, salt, and pepper. Cook for about 5 minutes, stirring often.

Stir in the BBQ sauce and simmer for an additional 5-10 minutes, or until thoroughly cooked and slightly thickened. Adjust the seasoning as needed.

While the mixture is cooking, toast the slider buns if desired. Place the BBQ pulled hearts of palm on the bottom half of each bread. Cover with coleslaw and the top half of the bread.

If preferred, garnish with fresh cilantro. Serve warm.

Eggplant "Meatballs" with Saffron Rice

Prep Time: 15 minutes

Cook Time: 30 minutes

Serving Size: 2 meatballs with 1 cup of rice (makes 4 servings)

(Per Serving):

Calories: 320

Carbs: 45g

Sugar: 3g

Protein: 10g

Fat: 12g

For the Eggplant Meatballs:

1 large eggplant (about 1 pound), diced

1/2 cup breadcrumbs (gluten-free if needed)

1/4 cup grated Parmesan cheese

1/4 cup chopped fresh parsley

2 cloves garlic, minced

1 teaspoon Italian seasoning

1/2 teaspoon salt

1/4 teaspoon black pepper

1 large egg, beaten

Olive oil for drizzling

For the Saffron Rice:

1 cup brown rice (or basmati rice)

2 cups water or low-sodium vegetable broth

1/4 teaspoon saffron threads

1 tablespoon olive oil

1/2 teaspoon salt

Zest of 1 lemon

Preheat the oven to 400 degrees Fahrenheit (200 degrees Celsius). Line a baking sheet with parchment paper.

Place the diced eggplant on a baking sheet, spray with olive oil, and roast for 20 minutes, or until tender and faintly caramelized.

In a large mixing bowl, combine the roasted eggplant, breadcrumbs, Parmesan cheese (if using), parsley, garlic, Italian seasoning, salt & pepper, and beaten egg. Mix until well mixed.

Shape the mixture into 1.5-inch meatballs and lay them back on the baking pan. Drizzle with a little more olive oil.

Continue baking in the preheated oven for 15-20 minutes, or until golden brown and firm.

While the meatballs bake, rinse the rice with cool water. Heat water or broth in a medium pot until it boils. Combine the saffron threads, olive oil, and salt. Add the rice, cover, and turn the heat to low. Cook for 40–45 minutes, or until the rice is cooked and the liquid has been absorbed. If preferred, season with lemon zest.

Plate the saffron rice and top with the eggplant "meatballs." Drizzle with more olive oil or your favorite sauce if preferred.

Tempeh and Sweet Potato Samosas

Prep Time: 20 minutes

Cook Time: 30 minutes

Serving Size: 2 samosas (makes 8 servings)

(Per Samosa):

Calories: 200

Carbs: 26g

Sugar: 2g

Protein: 6g

Fat: 9g

For the Filling:

1 medium sweet potato, peeled and diced (about 1 cup)

1 cup tempeh, crumbled

1 tablespoon olive oil

1/2 onion, finely chopped

2 cloves garlic, minced

1 teaspoon grated ginger

1 teaspoon ground cumin

1/2 teaspoon ground coriander

1/2 teaspoon turmeric powder

1/4 teaspoon cayenne pepper

1/2 teaspoon salt

1/4 teaspoon black pepper

1/2 cup frozen peas

For the Dough:

2 cups whole wheat flour (or gluten-free flour)

1/4 teaspoon salt

1/4 cup olive oil

1/4 cup cold water (more as needed)

In a mixing dish, add whole wheat flour and salt. Add the olive oil and combine until crumbly. Gradually add cold water until a smooth dough is formed. Knead for approximately 5 minutes, then cover and let sit for 20 minutes.

In a pan, heat the olive oil over medium heat. Sauté the chopped onion until transparent, approximately 5 minutes. Sauté for a further minute with the minced garlic and grated ginger. Add chopped sweet potatoes and a splash of water. Cover and simmer for about 10 minutes, or until the sweet potato is cooked.

Stir in the crumbled tempeh, cumin, coriander, turmeric, cayenne (if using), salt, and black pepper. Cook for a further 5 minutes, then add frozen peas if preferred. Take the filling off the stove and let it cool.

Divide the rested dough into eight equal parts. Roll each part into a ball and flatten into a circle approximately 6 inches in diameter. Cut the circle in half to get two semicircles. Take one semi-circle and fold the straight edge together to make a cone shape. Seal the edge with a little water. Fill the cone with the sweet potato-tempeh mixture, then close the open edge to make a triangle. Repeat with the remaining dough and filling.

Cook the samosas: The samosas may be baked or fried.

How to Bake: Preheat the oven to 400 °F (200 °C). Arrange the samosas on a baking sheet lined with parchment paper. Brush with olive oil and bake for 25–30 minutes, or until golden brown.

To fry: Heat the oil in a deep frying pan over medium heat. Fry the samosas in batches for about 4-5 minutes each side, or until golden and crispy. Drain onto paper towels.

Serve your Tempeh and Sweet Potato Samosas warm with your favorite chutney or yogurt for dipping.

Buffalo Cauliflower Tacos

Prep Time: 10 minutes

Cook Time: 25 minutes

Serving Size: 2 tacos (makes 4 servings)

(Per Taco):

Calories: 200

Carbs: 30g

Sugar: 1g

Protein: 5g

Fat: 8g

1 medium head of cauliflower, cut into florets

1 cup whole wheat flour (or gluten-free flour)

1 teaspoon garlic powder

1 teaspoon onion powder

1/2 teaspoon paprika

1/4 teaspoon salt

1/4 teaspoon black pepper

1/2 cup water

1/2 cup buffalo sauce (adjust to taste)

8 small corn or flour tortillas

1/2 cup shredded lettuce

1/2 avocado, sliced

Fresh cilantro, chopped

Lime wedges (for serving)

Set your oven to 425°F (220°C) and prepare a baking sheet with parchment paper.

In a large bowl, combine the flour, garlic powder, onion powder, paprika, salt, and black pepper. Gradually whisk in the water until the batter is smooth.

Dip the cauliflower florets into the batter, making sure they are well covered. Arrange the coated florets in a single layer on the prepared baking sheet.

Bake in a preheated oven for 20-25 minutes, or until soft and golden, turning halfway through to ensure equal cooking.

Once the cauliflower has finished roasting, take it from the oven and sprinkle it with buffalo sauce. Toss to coat well, then return to the oven for a further 5 minutes.

While the cauliflower bakes, cook the tortillas in a pan over medium heat for approximately 30 seconds on each side, or until flexible.

Fill the tortillas with buffalo cauliflower, shredded lettuce, and sliced avocado. Garnish with fresh cilantro.

Garnish your Buffalo Cauliflower Tacos with lime wedges for an added blast of flavor.

.

Portobello Wellington Bites

Prep Time: 15 minutes

Cook Time: 25 minutes

Serving Size: 2 bites (makes 4 servings)

(Per Bite):

Calories: 180

Carbs: 18g

Sugar: 1g

Protein: 5g

Fat: 10g

4 large portobello mushrooms, stems removed

1 sheet puff pastry (thawed if frozen)

1 cup cooked spinach, squeezed dry

1/2 cup ricotta cheese or a dairy-free alternative

1/4 cup grated Parmesan cheese (optional)

2 cloves garlic, minced

1 teaspoon dried thyme

1 teaspoon olive oil

Salt and pepper, to taste

1 egg (for egg wash, optional) or non-dairy milk (for a vegan option)

Preheat the oven to 400 degrees Fahrenheit (200 degrees Celsius). Line a baking sheet with parchment paper.

In a medium bowl, combine the cooked spinach, ricotta cheese, Parmesan cheese (if using), minced garlic, dried thyme, olive oil, salt, and pepper until thoroughly blended.

Place the portobello mushrooms, gills facing up, on the prepared baking sheet. Spread the spinach filling equally into each mushroom cap.

Roll out the puff pastry on a lightly floured board, then cut it into pieces big enough to cover each mushroom.

Place a puff pastry piece over each packed mushroom, pinching the edges to close. If desired, use a knife to cut a few slits on top to let steam escape.

If used, whip the egg and brush it across the puff pastry. For a vegan version, use non-dairy milk.

Bake in a preheated oven for 20-25 minutes, or until the crust is golden brown and puffy.

Allow the bites to cool for a few minutes before serving. Serve warm as an appetizer or small dinner.

Mediterranean Stuffed Artichokes

Prep Time: 15 minutes

Cook Time: 40 minutes

Serving Size: 1 stuffed artichoke (makes 4 servings)

(Per Stuffed Artichoke):

Calories: 220

Carbs: 28g

Sugar: 2g

Protein: 6g

Fat: 10g

- 4 medium artichokes
- 1 cup cooked quinoa (or brown rice)
- 1/2 cup cherry tomatoes, diced
- 1/4 cup black olives, pitted and chopped
- 1/4 cup red onion, finely chopped
- 1/4 cup fresh parsley, chopped
- 1/4 cup feta cheese, crumbled
- 2 tablespoons olive oil
- 1 tablespoon lemon juice
- 1 teaspoon dried oregano
- 1/2 teaspoon salt
- 1/4 teaspoon black pepper
- Lemon wedges

Preheat the oven to 375° Fahrenheit (190° Celsius). Trim the artichokes' stems and remove the tough outer leaves. Cut off the top of each artichoke about an inch from the top. Take a spoon and scrape out the fuzzy choke in the middle of each artichoke.

In a large mixing bowl, add cooked quinoa (or brown rice), diced cherry tomatoes, chopped olives, red onion, parsley, feta cheese (if using), olive oil, lemon juice, oregano, salt, and black pepper. Mix until well mixed.

Gently separate the leaves of each artichoke and push the filling mixture into them, pressing down to compress it in.

Place the filled artichokes in a baking dish with about an inch of water in the bottom. Cover with aluminum foil and bake for 30 minutes.

Remove the foil and bake for 10 more minutes, or until the artichokes are soft and the tops are brown.

Remove from the oven and let cool slightly. Serve warm, with lemon slices on the side.

Carrot "Lox" Bagel Stack

Prep Time: 15 minutes

Cook Time: 0 minutes

Serving Size: 1 stack (makes 2 servings)

(Per Stack):

Calories: 320

Carbs: 36g

Sugar: 3g

Protein: 8g

Fat: 15g

2 medium carrots, peeled and thinly sliced lengthwise (using a vegetable peeler or mandoline)

2 tablespoons tamari or soy sauce

1 tablespoon liquid smoke (optional)

2 whole-grain or gluten-free bagels

1/2 cup dairy-free cream cheese (or regular cream cheese)

1/2 avocado, sliced

1/4 red onion, thinly sliced

Fresh dill or chives for garnish

Capers for garnish

In a shallow bowl, mix together the tamari or soy sauce and liquid smoke (if using). Add the carrot slices and make sure they are completely covered. Allow them to marinade for a minimum of 10 minutes while you prepare the other ingredients.

As the carrots marinate, toast the bagels until golden brown.

Spread a liberal dollop of dairy-free cream cheese over each bagel half. Top with marinated carrots, avocado slices, and red onion.

Top with fresh dill or chives and, if wanted, capers.

Korean-Style Cauliflower Wings

Prep Time: 15 minutes

Cook Time: 30 minutes

Serving Size: 1 cup (makes 4 servings)

(Per Cup):

Calories: 180

Carbs: 16g

Sugar: 5g

Protein: 5g

Fat: 10g

1 medium head of cauliflower, cut into florets

1/2 cup almond flour (or gluten-free flour)

1/2 cup water

1 teaspoon garlic powder

1 teaspoon onion powder

1/2 teaspoon salt

1/4 teaspoon black pepper

1/2 cup Korean BBQ sauce (check for low-sugar options or make your own)

1 tablespoon sesame oil

Sesame seeds

Green onions, chopped

Set your oven to 425°F (220°C). Line a baking sheet with parchment paper.

In a large mixing bowl, combine almond flour, water, garlic powder, onion powder, salt, and black pepper. Whisk until smooth.

Dip each cauliflower floret in the batter, letting the excess fall off. Spread the coated florets out on the prepared baking sheet in a single layer.

Place the cauliflower in a preheated oven for 25-30 minutes, or until golden brown and crispy. Flip halfway through.

In a small saucepan, heat the Korean BBQ sauce and sesame oil over low heat until heated. Once the cauliflower has finished roasting, mix it in the heated sauce until well covered.

Place the sauced cauliflower wings on a serving plate and decorate with sesame seeds and chopped green onions. Serve immediately.

.

Green Tea Soba Noodle Pancakes

Prep Time: 10 minutes

Cook Time: 15 minutes

Serving Size: 2 pancakes (makes 4 servings)

(Per Pancake):

Calories: 150

Carbs: 18g

Sugar: 1g

Protein: 6g

Fat: 7g

1 cup cooked soba noodles

2 large eggs

1 tablespoon matcha green tea powder

1/4 cup grated zucchini (squeezed to remove excess moisture)

1/4 cup finely chopped green onions

1/4 teaspoon salt

1/4 teaspoon black pepper

2 tablespoons sesame oil or olive oil for cooking

sliced avocado, soy sauce, or tahini

In a large mixing bowl, combine cooked soba noodles, eggs, matcha powder, shredded zucchini, sliced green onions, salt, and black pepper. Mix until well mixed. The mixture should be somewhat thickened.

In a nonstick pan, heat 1 tablespoon sesame oil over medium heat.

Pour half of the noodle mixture onto the skillet and shape it into a pancake. Cook for about 3-4 minutes each side, or until golden brown and crispy. Repeat with the entire mixture, using more oil as required.

Serve the pancakes warm, topped with sliced avocado and drizzled with soy sauce or tahini, as preferred.

Crispy Quinoa and Vegetable Fritters

Prep Time: 15 minutes

Cook Time: 20 minutes

Serving Size: 2 fritters (makes 4 servings)

(Per Fritter):

Calories: 120

Carbs: 15g

Sugar: 1g

Protein: 4g

Fat: 5g

- 1 cup cooked quinoa
- 1 cup grated zucchini about 1 medium zucchini
- 1/2 cup grated carrot about 1 medium carrot
- 1/2 cup finely chopped bell pepper (any color)
- 2 large eggs
- 1/4 cup almond flour or whole wheat flour
- 1 teaspoon garlic powder
- 1/2 teaspoon cumin
- 1/4 teaspoon salt
- 1/4 teaspoon black pepper
- 2 tablespoons olive oil (for frying)
- Fresh herbs (like parsley or cilantro) for garnish

In a large mixing bowl, add cooked quinoa, grated zucchini, grated carrot, diced bell pepper, eggs, almond flour, garlic powder, cumin, salt, and black pepper. Mix until well mixed.

With your hands, shape the mixture into little patties approximately 2-3 inches in diameter.

Heat the olive oil in a large pan over medium heat. Once heated, add the fritters in batches, taking care not to overcrowd the pan. Cook for about 3-4 minutes each side, or until golden brown and crispy.

Once cooked, place the fritters on a paper towel-lined platter to absorb any leftover oil.

Top with fresh herbs if wanted and serve warm. These fritters go well with a yogurt or avocado dip.

Roasted Grape and Fig Flatbread

Prep Time: 10 minutes

Cook Time: 20 minutes

Serving Size: 1 flatbread (makes 2 servings)

(Per Serving):

Calories: 290

Carbs: 42g

Sugar: 10g

Protein: 8g

Fat: 10g

1 cup seedless grapes (red or green)

4 fresh figs, sliced or 1/2 cup dried figs

1 tablespoon olive oil

1 teaspoon balsamic vinegar

1 teaspoon fresh thyme leaves or 1/2 teaspoon dried thyme

Salt and black pepper to taste

1 whole grain flatbread or pita

1/4 cup goat cheese or feta cheese

Fresh arugula for topping

Preheat the oven to 400 degrees Fahrenheit (200 degrees Celsius). Line a baking sheet with parchment paper.

In a bowl, combine the grapes, olive oil, balsamic vinegar, thyme, salt, and pepper. Spread the grapes evenly on the prepared baking sheet. Roast for about 15 minutes, or until the grapes are tender and slightly caramelized.

While the grapes roast, set the flatbread on a baking sheet. If using goat or feta cheese, evenly distribute it on the flatbread.

Once the grapes have been roasted, take them from the oven and put the sliced figs and roasted grapes on the flatbread.

Return the flatbread to the oven and bake for another 5-7 minutes, or until crispy and the cheese (if using) is melted.

Remove the flatbread from the oven and allow it to cool slightly. If desired, top with freshly chopped arugula. Slice and serve warm.

Pistachio-Crusted Tofu Cutlets

Prep Time: 15 minutes

Cook Time: 25 minutes

Serving Size: 1 cutlet (makes 4 servings)

(Per Cutlet):

Calories: 210

Carbohydrates: 12g

Sugar: 1g

Protein: 11g

Fat: 15g

1 block (14 oz) firm or extra-firm tofu, drained and pressed

1 cup shelled pistachios

1/2 cup breadcrumbs (gluten-free if needed)

1 tablespoon olive oil

1 teaspoon garlic powder

1 teaspoon onion powder

1/2 teaspoon salt

1/4 teaspoon black pepper

2 tablespoons nutritional yeast

2 tablespoons Dijon mustard or vegan mayo (for coating)

Preheat the oven to 400 degrees Fahrenheit (200 degrees Celsius). Line a baking sheet with parchment paper.

Cut the pressed tofu into half-inch thick cutlets.

In a food processor, mix pistachios, breadcrumbs, garlic powder, onion powder, salt, black pepper, and nutritional yeast (if using). Pulse the ingredients until they resemble coarse crumbs.

Brush each tofu cutlet with Dijon mustard or vegan mayonnaise. Then, push each cutlet into the pistachio mixture, making sure it's well covered on both sides.

Arrange the coated tofu cutlets on the prepared baking sheet. Drizzle with olive oil. Bake in a preheated oven for 20-25 minutes, turning halfway through, or until golden brown and crispy.

Serve the pistachio-crusted tofu cutlets warm, with a side salad or steaming veggies.

Millet and Vegetable Hand Pies

Prep Time: 15 minutes

Cook Time: 30 minutes

Serving Size: 1 pie (makes 8 servings)

(Per Pie):

Calories: 230

Carbs: 35g

Sugar: 2g

Protein: 6g

Fat: 8g

For the Filling:

1 cup cooked millet (about 1/2 cup dry)

1 cup diced mixed vegetables (such as carrots, peas, and bell peppers)

1/2 cup chopped spinach or kale

1 tablespoon olive oil

1 teaspoon garlic powder

1 teaspoon onion powder

1/2 teaspoon salt

1/4 teaspoon black pepper

For the Dough:

2 cups whole wheat flour (or gluten-free flour)

1/2 teaspoon salt

1/2 cup cold olive oil or coconut oil

6-8 tablespoons cold water

In a pan, heat the olive oil over medium heat. Combine the chopped mixed veggies with garlic powder, onion powder, salt, and black pepper. Sauté the veggies for around 5-7 minutes, until they are soft. Stir in the cooked millet and chopped spinach. Remove from heat and let cool.

In a large mixing basin, combine whole wheat flour and salt. Add the cold oil and combine until crumbly. Gradually add cold water, 1 tablespoon at a time, and mix until dough forms. Knead lightly till smooth, then cover and let sit for 10 minutes.

Set the oven to 375°F (190°C) and line a baking sheet with parchment paper.

On a floured surface, roll out the dough to approximately 1/8 inch thickness. Cut into six-inch rounds. Put 1-2 teaspoons of the millet and vegetable mixture in the middle of each round. Fold the dough over to form a half-moon shape, then flatten the edges with a fork.

Arrange the hand pies on the prepared baking sheet. Bake for 25–30 minutes, or until golden brown.

Let the hand pies cool slightly before serving. Enjoy warmth as a snack or supper.

Stuffed King Oyster Mushroom "Scallops"

Prep Time: 15 minutes

Cook Time: 25 minutes

Serving Size: 2 "scallops" (makes 4 servings)

(Per "Scallop"):

Calories: 120

Carbs: 18g

Sugar: 1g

Protein: 5g

Fat: 4g

- 2 large king oyster mushrooms
- 1 cup cooked quinoa
- 1/4 cup diced red bell pepper
- 1/4 cup finely chopped green onions
- 2 cloves garlic, minced
- 1 tablespoon olive oil
- 1 teaspoon lemon juice
- 1 teaspoon dried thyme
- 1/2 teaspoon salt
- 1/4 teaspoon black pepper
- 1/4 cup nutritional yeast
- Fresh parsley, chopped (for garnish)

Set the oven to 375°F (190°C) and line a baking sheet with parchment paper.

Clean the king oyster mushrooms and cut into 1-inch-thick "scallops." Using a tiny spoon, carefully hollow out the middle of each mushroom slice, leaving a small hole for the filling.

Heat olive oil in a pan over medium heat, then sauté minced garlic for 1-2 minutes, until fragrant. Cook for a further 3-4 minutes, or until the diced red bell pepper and green onions soften. Add the cooked quinoa, lemon juice, dried thyme, salt, black pepper, and nutritional yeast (if desired). Mix well and remove from heat.

Place the quinoa mixture in the hollowed-out mushrooms, packing them gently.

Transfer the filled mushrooms to the prepared baking sheet and bake for 20-25 minutes, or until soft and slightly brown.

Remove from the oven, sprinkle with chopped fresh parsley, and eat warm.

SOUPS AND STEWS

Moroccan Harissa Lentil Stew

Prep Time: 10 minutes

Cook Time: 30 minutes

Serving Size: 1 cup (makes 4 servings)

(Per Cup):

Calories: 210

Carbs: 36g

Sugar: 4g

Protein: 12g

Fat: 4g

- 1 cup green or brown lentils, rinsed
- 1 tablespoon olive oil
- 1 medium onion, diced
- 2 cloves garlic, minced
- 1 medium carrot, diced
- 1 medium bell pepper, diced
- 1 can (14.5 oz) diced tomatoes
- 4 cups vegetable broth or water
- 2 tablespoons harissa paste (adjust for spice preference)
- 1 teaspoon ground cumin
- 1 teaspoon ground coriander
- 1/2 teaspoon salt
- 1/4 teaspoon black pepper
- 1 cup chopped kale or spinach
- Fresh cilantro or parsley for garnish
- Lemon wedges for serving

To sauté the vegetables, heat olive oil in a large saucepan over medium heat. Sauté the chopped onion and garlic for 3-4 minutes, until softened.

Stir in the carrot and bell pepper and simmer for another 5 minutes, or until softened.

Add the rinsed lentils, chopped tomatoes (including juice), vegetable broth, harissa paste, cumin, coriander, salt, and black pepper. Stir to mix.

Bring the stew to a boil, then turn the heat down to low. Cover and simmer for about 25 minutes, or until the lentils are cooked. If using, add the chopped kale or spinach during the last 5 minutes of cooking.

Taste the stew and adjust seasoning as needed. If it's too thick, add some additional broth or water.

Ladle the stew into bowls, top with fresh cilantro or parsley, and serve with lemon wedges on the side to squeeze.

Miso Mushroom & Kelp Soup

Prep Time: 10 minutes

Cook Time: 15 minutes

Serving Size: 1 cup (makes 4 servings)

(Per Cup):

Calories: 80

Carbs: 10g

Sugar: 2g

Protein: 6g

Fat: 3g

- 4 cups vegetable broth or water
- 1 cup sliced mushrooms (shiitake or cremini)
- 1/4 cup dried kelp (kombu), soaked in water for 10 minutes and sliced
- 2 tablespoons miso paste (white or yellow)
- 1 cup diced tofu (firm or silken)
- 2 green onions, sliced
- 1 teaspoon grated fresh ginger
- 1 teaspoon sesame oil
- 1/2 cup baby spinach or bok choy
- Sea salt to taste

In a large saucepan, boil the vegetable broth or water to a moderate simmer over medium heat.

Place the sliced mushrooms, soaked and sliced kelp, diced tofu, grated ginger, and sesame oil in the saucepan. Simmer for 5-7 minutes, until the mushrooms are soft.

In a small bowl, mix together the miso paste with a ladle of heated soup until smooth. Stir the miso mixture back into the saucepan. To maintain the beneficial bacteria included in miso, avoid boiling the soup after adding it.

If using, mix in the baby spinach or bok choy and simmer for another 2-3 minutes, until wilted.

Remove from heat, season with sea salt to taste, and garnish with sliced green onions. Serve hot.

Brazilian Fish Stew (Moqueca)

Prep Time: 15 minutes

Cook Time: 30 minutes

Serving Size: 1 cup (makes 4 servings)

(Per Cup):

Calories: 290

Carbs: 14g

Sugar: 2g

Protein: 24g

Fat: 18g

1 lb (450g) white fish filets (such as cod, tilapia, or snapper), cut into chunks

1 tablespoon lime juice

1/2 teaspoon salt

1/2 teaspoon black pepper

1 tablespoon olive oil

1 medium onion, chopped

4 cloves garlic, minced

1 bell pepper (any color), chopped

2 medium tomatoes, chopped

1 can (14 oz) coconut milk

1/4 cup fresh cilantro, chopped (plus more for garnish)

1 teaspoon paprika

1 teaspoon turmeric

1/2 teaspoon cayenne pepper

In a dish, mix the fish pieces with lime juice, salt, and black pepper. Allow it to marinade for approximately 10 minutes.

To sauté vegetables, heat olive oil in a large saucepan over medium heat. Add the chopped onion and cook for approximately 5 minutes, or until transparent. Cook for a further 5 minutes, adding the minced garlic, bell pepper, and chopped tomatoes until the veggies soften.

Mix in the paprika, turmeric, and cayenne pepper (if using) until thoroughly combined with the veggies.

Add the coconut milk and bring the mixture to a boil. Add the marinated fish pieces and simmer for 10-15 minutes, or until the fish is cooked through and easily flaked with a fork.

Stir in the chopped cilantro, leaving a bit for decoration. Taste and adjust seasoning as needed.

Ladle the stew into dishes and sprinkle with more cilantro if desired. Serve warm, preferably with brown rice or quinoa..

Green Detox Soup

Prep Time: 10 minutes

Cook Time: 20 minutes

Serving Size: 1 cup (makes 4 servings)

(Per Cup):

Calories: 180

Carbs: 18g

Sugar: 3g

Protein: 6g

Fat: 10g

- 1 tablespoon olive oil
- 1 medium onion, chopped
- 2 cloves garlic, minced
- 4 cups vegetable broth (low-sodium)
- 2 cups chopped kale or spinach
- 2 medium zucchini, diced
- 1 cup green peas (fresh or frozen)
- 1 medium cucumber, peeled and diced
- 1 avocado, pitted and diced
- 1/4 cup fresh parsley, chopped
- 1 tablespoon lemon juice
- Salt and black pepper to taste
- Pumpkin seeds or hemp seeds for garnish

Warm olive oil in a large saucepan over medium heat. Add the chopped onion and cook for approximately 5 minutes, or until transparent. Sauté the minced garlic for another minute, until aromatic.

Add the veggie broth and bring to a boil. Combine the chopped kale or spinach, diced zucchini, and green peas. Reduce the heat to a simmer and cook for 10-15 minutes, or until the veggies are soft.

Remove the saucepan from the heat. Using an immersion blender, purée the soup until smooth. Alternatively, put the soup to a blender and process in batches until smooth.

Return the pureed soup to the pot (if you used a blender). Combine the chopped cucumber, avocado, fresh parsley, and lemon juice. Season with salt and black pepper to taste.

Ladle the soup into dishes and top with optional pumpkin or hemp seeds.

Golden Bone Broth Soup with Root Vegetables

Prep Time: 10 minutes

Cook Time: 1 hour 30 minutes

Serving Size: 1 cup (makes 4 servings)

(Per Cup):

Calories: 150

Carbs: 20g

Sugar: 3g

Protein: 6g

Fat: 5g

4 cups bone broth (homemade or store-bought)

2 medium carrots, diced

2 medium parsnips, diced

1 medium sweet potato, diced

1 cup chopped celery

1/2 onion, diced

3 cloves garlic, minced

1 tablespoon olive oil

1 teaspoon turmeric powder

1/2 teaspoon dried thyme

1/2 teaspoon salt

1/4 teaspoon black pepper

Fresh parsley, chopped

To sauté the vegetables, heat olive oil in a large saucepan over medium heat. Sauté the chopped onion and minced garlic for 2-3 minutes, until aromatic.

Combine the chopped carrots, parsnips, sweet potato, and celery. Sauté for 5 more minutes, stirring periodically.

Pour in the bone broth and season with turmeric, dried thyme, salt, and black pepper. Heat the mixture to a boil.

Once the soup has boiled, decrease the heat to low and let it simmer for approximately an hour, or until the veggies are soft.

Ladle the soup into dishes and top with fresh parsley, if preferred. Serve it warm as a nutritious dinner.

Persian Pomegranate Walnut Stew (Fesenjan)

Prep Time: 15 minutes

Cook Time: 1 hour 30 minutes

Serving Size: 1 cup (makes 4 servings)

(Per Cup):

Calories: 400

Carbs: 14g

Sugar: 5g

Protein: 24g

Fat: 30g

1 pound chicken thighs or drumsticks (bone-in, skinless)

2 cups walnuts, finely ground

2 medium onions, finely chopped

2 cups pomegranate juice (unsweetened)

1 tablespoon olive oil

1 teaspoon turmeric powder

1/2 teaspoon cinnamon

1/4 teaspoon salt

1/4 teaspoon black pepper

1 tablespoon maple syrup or honey

Pomegranate seeds

Fresh parsley or cilantro

Heat the olive oil in a big saucepan or Dutch oven over medium heat. Sauté the chopped onions until transparent, approximately 5 minutes. Cook the chicken thighs until browned on both sides, approximately 5-7 minutes.

Combine turmeric, cinnamon, salt, and black pepper. Stir in the finely ground walnuts and simmer for another 2 minutes, stirring regularly.

Pour the pomegranate juice into the mixture and bring to a boil. Reduce the heat to low, cover, and let simmer for approximately an hour, stirring periodically. If the stew gets too thick, add more water to achieve the appropriate consistency.

For a sweeter stew, add maple syrup or honey in the final 10 minutes of simmering.

Once the chicken is cooked and the flavors have combined, remove from the fire. Serve the stew in dishes topped with pomegranate seeds and fresh herbs.

Thai Coconut Kabocha Squash Soup

Prep Time: 10 minutes

Cook Time: 30 minutes

Serving Size: 1 cup (makes 4 servings)

(Per Cup):

Calories: 240

Carbs: 18g

Sugar: 4g

Protein: 4g

Fat: 18g

1 medium kabocha squash (about 2-3 cups, peeled and cubed)

1 tablespoon coconut oil

1 medium onion, diced

3 cloves garlic, minced

1 tablespoon fresh ginger, minced

1 can (13.5 oz) coconut milk

3 cups vegetable broth

1 tablespoon red curry paste (adjust to taste)

1 tablespoon soy sauce or tamari (for gluten-free)

Juice of 1 lime

Salt and pepper to taste

Fresh cilantro, chopped (for garnish)

Sliced red chili, toasted coconut flakes, or green onions

In a big saucepan, heat the coconut oil over medium heat. Add the chopped onion and cook for 5-7 minutes, or until transparent. Cook for a further 1-2 minutes, stirring in the minced garlic and ginger until fragrant.

Place the diced kabocha squash in the saucepan, followed by the vegetable broth and red curry paste. Bring to a boil and then lower to a simmer. Cook for 15 to 20 minutes, or until the squash is soft.

When the squash is cooked, remove the saucepan from the heat. Puree the soup with an immersion blender until smooth, or transfer it to a countertop blender in stages.

Return the pureed soup to the pot (if you used a countertop blender). Stir in the coconut milk, soy sauce (or tamari), lime juice, salt, and pepper. Heat gently until warmed through.

Pour the soup into dishes and sprinkle with chopped cilantro and any other toppings you choose..

Black Sesame & Purple Sweet Potato Stew

Prep Time: 15 minutes

Cook Time: 30 minutes

Serving Size: 1 bowl (makes 4 servings)

(Per Bowl):

Calories: 280

Carbs: 40g

Sugar: 6g

Protein: 8g

Fat: 10g

2 medium purple sweet potatoes, peeled and diced (about 2 cups)

1 cup black sesame paste (tahini can be used as a substitute)

4 cups vegetable broth (low-sodium)

1 cup diced carrots

1 cup chopped kale or spinach

1/2 cup chopped onions

3 cloves garlic, minced

1 tablespoon ginger, grated

2 tablespoons soy sauce or tamari (for gluten-free)

1 tablespoon olive oil

1/2 teaspoon turmeric powder

1/4 teaspoon black pepper

Fresh cilantro or green onions for garnish

To sauté the vegetables, heat olive oil in a large saucepan over medium heat. Sauté the chopped onions, garlic, and ginger until they are transparent (approximately 3-4 minutes).

Combine the chopped purple sweet potatoes and carrots. Cook for a further 5 minutes, stirring occasionally.

Add the vegetable broth, black sesame paste, turmeric powder, and black pepper. Bring to a boil, then decrease heat and let simmer for 15-20 minutes, or until the sweet potatoes are cooked.

Combine the chopped kale or spinach with the soy sauce or tamari. Cook for another 5 minutes, until the greens have wilted.

Ladle the stew into dishes and top with fresh cilantro or green onions, if preferred.

Ethiopian Red Lentil Stew (Misir Wat)

Prep Time: 10 minutes

Cook Time: 30 minutes

Serving Size: 1 cup (makes 4 servings)

(Per Cup):

Calories: 210

Carbs: 34g

Sugar: 4g

Protein: 12g

Fat: 5g

1 cup red lentils, rinsed and drained

1 medium onion, finely chopped

2 cloves garlic, minced

1 tablespoon ginger, grated

2 tablespoons olive oil

2 tablespoons berbere spice blend (adjust to taste)

2 cups vegetable broth or water

1 can (14 oz) diced tomatoes (with juices)

1/2 teaspoon salt or to taste

1/4 teaspoon black pepper

1 tablespoon lemon juice (for serving)

Fresh cilantro or parsley for garnish

In a large saucepan, heat the olive oil over medium heat. Sauté the chopped onion for 5-7 minutes, until transparent. Stir in the minced garlic and grated ginger, simmering for another 1-2 minutes until aromatic.

Stir in the berbere spice combination and heat for another minute to unleash the flavors.

Place the washed red lentils, chopped tomatoes (with juices), vegetable broth, salt, and black pepper in a saucepan. Bring to a boil, then turn the heat down to low. Simmer uncovered for 20-25 minutes, stirring periodically, until the lentils are cooked and the stew thickens. If it gets too thick, add a little more water or broth.

Once done, add lemon juice to brighten. Season with extra salt and pepper as required.

Serve warm with fresh cilantro or parsley, and top with injera or rice..

Japanese Ginger & Daikon Soup

Prep Time: 10 minutes

Cook Time: 20 minutes

Serving Size: 1 cup (makes 4 servings)

(Per Cup):

Calories: 80

Carbs: 12g

Sugar: 2g

Protein: 3g

Fat: 3g

1 tablespoon sesame oil

1 small onion, diced

2 cloves garlic, minced

1 tablespoon fresh ginger, grated

2 cups daikon radish, peeled and diced (about 1 medium daikon)

4 cups low-sodium vegetable broth or water

2 cups chopped bok choy or spinach

1 tablespoon soy sauce or tamari (for gluten-free)

1 teaspoon rice vinegar

Salt and pepper to taste

Green onions, sliced

Warm sesame oil in a large saucepan over medium heat. Add the chopped onion and cook for approximately 5 minutes, or until transparent. Sauté the minced garlic and grated ginger for a further minute, or until fragrant.

Add the diced daikon radish and simmer for a further 5 minutes, stirring periodically.

Pour in the veggie broth or water and bring to a boil. Reduce the heat to a simmer for approximately 10 minutes, or until the daikon is soft.

Combine chopped bok choy or spinach, soy sauce, and rice vinegar. Simmer for another 2-3 minutes, until the greens have wilted. Season with salt and pepper to taste.

Ladle the soup into dishes, top with chopped green onions.

MEAT, SEAFOOD, POULTRY AND OTHER PROTEINS

Turmeric-Ginger Poached Sea Bass with Saffron Broth

Prep Time: 10 minutes

Cook Time: 20 minutes

Serving Size: 1 filet (makes 2 servings)

(Per Fillet):

Calories: 280

Carbs: 5g

Sugar: 1g

Protein: 30g

Fat: 15g

2 (6-ounce) sea bass filets

2 cups low-sodium vegetable broth

1 cup water

1 teaspoon turmeric powder

1 tablespoon grated fresh ginger

1/4 teaspoon saffron threads

1 tablespoon olive oil

1/2 teaspoon salt

1/4 teaspoon black pepper

Fresh lemon wedges (for serving)

Fresh cilantro or parsley

In a medium saucepan, whisk together vegetable broth, water, turmeric powder, grated ginger, saffron threads, salt, and black pepper. Bring to a moderate simmer over medium heat.

Once the stock is boiling, gently add the sea bass filets. Cover the pot and poach the fish for 8-10 minutes, or until it flakes easily with a fork and is well cooked.

Carefully take the sea bass from the soup and transfer it to serving dishes. Drizzle with olive oil and ladle saffron broth over the fish.

Serve with fresh lemon wedges and optional cilantro or parsley.

Mackerel En Papillote with Green Tea and Citrus

Prep Time: 10 minutes

Cook Time: 20 minutes

Serving Size: 1 filet (makes 2 servings)

(Per Fillet):

Calories: 220

Carbs: 6g

Sugar: 2g

Protein: 22g

Fat: 12g

2 mackerel filets

1 green tea bag

1 cup boiling water

1 orange, thinly sliced

1 lemon, thinly sliced

1 tablespoon olive oil

1 teaspoon fresh ginger, grated

1/2 teaspoon salt

1/4 teaspoon black pepper

Fresh herbs (like dill or parsley) for garnish

Set your oven to 375°F (190°C).

Steep the green tea bag in 1 cup boiling water for 3-5 minutes. Remove the tea bag and let it cool slightly.

Cut two big sheets of parchment paper (approximately 12x16 inches) into packages for the fish.

Place one mackerel filet on one side of each parchment paper. Drizzle with olive oil and garnish with grated ginger, salt, and black pepper. Place orange and lemon slices on top of the filet, then sprinkle with some of the brewed green tea.

Fold the remaining half of the parchment paper over the fish and crimp the edges securely to seal the package fully.

Place the packets on a baking sheet and bake in a preheated oven for 15-20 minutes, or until the fish is well cooked and readily flaked with a fork.

Carefully open the packets (avoid steam) and garnish with fresh herbs if desired. Serve with your preferred side, such as steamed veggies or rice.

Duck Breast with Tart Cherry Reduction

Prep Time: 10 minutes

Cook Time: 25 minutes

Serving Size: 1 duck breast (makes 2 servings)

(Per Serving):

Calories: 350

Carbs: 20g

Sugar: 15g

Protein: 25g

Fat: 20g

2 duck breasts

Salt and black pepper, to taste

1 cup tart cherry juice (unsweetened)

1 tablespoon honey or maple syrup (optional)

1 tablespoon balsamic vinegar

1 teaspoon fresh thyme leaves or 1/2 teaspoon dried thyme

1 tablespoon olive oil

Score the skin of each duck breast in a crisscross pattern, taking care not to cut into the flesh. Season both sides with salt and black pepper.

Place the duck breasts skin-side down in a pan over medium heat. Cook for 6-8 minutes, or until the fat renders and the skin is crispy. Flip the duck breasts and cook for another 4-6 minutes, or until the internal temperature reaches 135°F (57°C) for medium-rare. Remove the duck from the pan and set aside for 5 minutes before slicing.

In the same skillet, drain the excess grease, leaving approximately 1 tbsp. Combine the tart cherry juice, honey or maple syrup (if using), balsamic vinegar, and thyme. Bring to a boil, then decrease heat and simmer for 10-15 minutes, stirring regularly, until the sauce has thickened somewhat.

Slice the duck breast and place it on plates. Drizzle with tart cherry reduction.

To finish the dish, serve with steamed vegetables or a salad.

Sardine and Anchovy Puttanesca

Prep Time: 10 minutes

Cook Time: 15 minutes

Serving Size: 1 cup (makes 2 servings)

(Per Serving):

Calories: 320

Carbs: 45g

Sugar: 4g

Protein: 15g

Fat: 12g

- 8 ounces whole grain spaghetti or gluten-free pasta
- 2 tablespoons olive oil
- 2 cloves garlic, minced
- 1 can (15 ounces) diced tomatoes (with juice)
- 1 can (4-6 ounces) sardines in olive oil, drained and chopped
- 4-6 anchovy filets, chopped
- 1/4 cup black olives, pitted and sliced
- 1 teaspoon red pepper flakes (adjust to taste)
- 1 teaspoon dried oregano
- Salt and black pepper to taste
- Fresh parsley, chopped

In a large pot of salted boiling water, cook the spaghetti according to package directions until al dente. Drain the pasta and put aside, leaving 1/2 cup of the water.

In a large pan over medium heat, combine the olive oil and minced garlic. Sauté for approximately a minute, until aromatic, taking care not to burn the garlic.

Add the diced tomatoes (with liquid), chopped sardines, anchovy filets, olives, red pepper flakes, oregano, salt, and black pepper. Simmer for 5-7 minutes to let the flavors mingle.

Toss the cooked spaghetti in the skillet. If the sauce is too thick, add some of the remaining pasta water until it reaches the appropriate consistency.

Divide the pasta between two dishes, garnish with fresh parsley, and serve your Sardine and Anchovy Puttanesca warm..

Mussels in Golden Milk Broth

Prep Time: 10 minutes

Cook Time: 15 minutes

Serving Size: 1 cup mussels with broth (makes 2 servings)

(Per Serving):

Calories: 340

Carbs: 10g

Sugar: 2g

Protein: 22g

Fat: 25g

- 1 pound fresh mussels, cleaned and debearded
- 1 tablespoon olive oil
- 2 cloves garlic, minced
- 1 teaspoon fresh ginger, grated
- 1 teaspoon turmeric powder
- 1/2 teaspoon cumin
- 1/4 teaspoon cayenne pepper
- 1 can (14 oz) coconut milk
- 1 cup vegetable broth (low-sodium)
- Juice of 1 lime
- Salt and pepper, to taste
- Fresh cilantro or parsley, for garnish

In a large saucepan, warm the olive oil over medium heat. Sauté the minced garlic and grated ginger for approximately 1-2 minutes, until aromatic.

Stir in the turmeric, cumin, and cayenne pepper (if using) and simmer for another 30 seconds.

Pour the coconut milk and vegetable broth into the saucepan. Bring to a simmer.

After the stock has simmered, add the cleaned mussels. Cover the saucepan and boil for 5-7 minutes, or until the mussels are open. Discard any that remain closed.

Remove from heat, mix in lime juice, and season with salt and pepper as desired. Ladle the mussels and liquid into dishes, then garnish with fresh cilantro or parsley.

Grass-fed Liver with Rosemary and Blueberry Compote

Prep Time: 15 minutes

Cook Time: 15 minutes

Serving Size: 4 ounces liver with 2 tablespoons compote (makes 2 servings)

(Per Serving):

Calories: 350

Carbs: 20g

Sugar: 10g

Protein: 40g

Fat: 15g

For the Liver:

8 ounces grass-fed liver, sliced into 1/2-inch pieces

2 tablespoons olive oil

1 teaspoon fresh rosemary, chopped or 1/2 teaspoon dried rosemary

1/2 teaspoon salt

1/4 teaspoon black pepper

For the Blueberry Compote:

1 cup fresh or frozen blueberries

1 tablespoon honey or maple syrup (optional)

1 teaspoon lemon juice

1 teaspoon fresh rosemary, chopped or 1/2 teaspoon dried rosemary

In a small saucepan over medium heat, mix the blueberries, honey or maple syrup (if using), lemon juice, and rosemary. Cook for 5–7 minutes, stirring regularly, until the blueberries burst and the sauce thickens. Remove from the heat and put aside.

In a pan, heat the olive oil over medium-high heat. Season the liver slices with salt, black pepper, and fresh rosemary. Cook the liver in the pan for 3-4 minutes each side, or until browned and cooked through but still slightly pink in the middle.

Plate the cooked liver and top with the blueberry compote.

If preferred, serve with extra fresh rosemary on top.

Broiled Quail with Green Tea Rub

Prep Time: 15 minutes

Cook Time: 15 minutes

Serving Size: 1 quail (makes 4 servings)

(Per Quail):

Calories: 180

Carbs: 1g

Sugar: 0g

Protein: 25g

Fat: 8g

4 quail, cleaned and prepared

2 tablespoons green tea leaves (or 2 green tea bags)

1 tablespoon olive oil

1 teaspoon garlic powder

1 teaspoon onion powder

1 teaspoon smoked paprika

1/2 teaspoon salt

1/4 teaspoon black pepper

1 tablespoon fresh lemon juice

Fresh herbs (like parsley or thyme) for garnish

In a small bowl, mix together the green tea leaves, olive oil, garlic powder, onion powder, smoked paprika, salt, and black pepper. Combine until it forms a paste.

Pat the quail dry with paper towels. Rub the green tea mixture over the quail, being careful to coat them evenly. Allow them to marinade for at least 10 minutes.

Turn your oven's broiler to high and position a rack approximately 6 inches from the heat source.

Transfer the marinated fowl to a broiler-safe pan or baking sheet. Broil the quail for approximately 5-7 minutes each side, or until fully cooked and golden. Internal temperature should be 165°F (74°C).

Once done, take the quail out of the oven and sprinkle it with fresh lemon juice

Top with fresh herbs if wanted and serve warm..

Black Cod Misoyaki with Wasabi Greens

Prep Time: 15 minutes

Cook Time: 15 minutes

Serving Size: 1 filet with greens (makes 2 servings)

(Per Serving):

Calories: 350

Carbs: 15g

Sugar: 3g

Protein: 30g

Fat: 20g

For the Black Cod Misoyaki:

2 black cod filets (about 6 ounces each)

1/4 cup white miso paste

2 tablespoons sake or rice vinegar

2 tablespoons mirin or honey

1 tablespoon soy sauce or tamari for gluten-free

For the Wasabi Greens:

4 cups mixed greens (such as kale, spinach, or arugula)

1 teaspoon wasabi paste (adjust to taste)

1 tablespoon olive oil

1 teaspoon sesame oil

1 tablespoon rice vinegar

Salt and pepper to taste

In a basin, mix together the miso paste, sake, mirin, and soy sauce to prepare the marinade. Marinate the black cod filets for at least 30 minutes before refrigerating.

Preheat the oven to 400 °F (200 °C). Remove the fish from the marinade, allowing excess marinade to drop off. Put the filets on a baking sheet lined with parchment paper. Bake for 12-15 minutes, or until the fish is flaky and cooked thoroughly.

While the fish cooks, combine the wasabi paste, olive oil, sesame oil, rice vinegar, salt, and pepper in a big dish. Toss in the mixed greens until uniformly coated.

Place the wasabi greens on two dishes. Top with the roasted black cod filets. Drizzle the leftover sauce from the baking sheet over the fish to add flavor.

Venison Medallions with Pomegranate Glaze

Prep Time: 10 minutes

Cook Time: 15 minutes

Serving Size: 4 medallions (makes 2 servings)

(Per Serving):

Calories: 320

Carbs: 18g

Sugar: 12g

Protein: 30g

Fat: 14g

1 pound venison tenderloin, cut into 1-inch medallions

1/2 teaspoon salt

1/2 teaspoon black pepper

1 tablespoon olive oil

1/2 cup pomegranate juice

2 tablespoons honey or maple syrup for a refined-sugar-free option

1 tablespoon balsamic vinegar

1 teaspoon fresh rosemary, chopped or 1/2 teaspoon dried rosemary

Fresh pomegranate seeds

Rub the venison medallions with salt and black pepper on both sides.

To sear the medallions, heat olive oil in a large pan over medium-high heat. Add the venison medallions and sear for 3-4 minutes each side, or until browned and cooked to your preferred doneness. Remove from the skillet and put aside.

In the same pan, combine the pomegranate juice, honey, balsamic vinegar, and rosemary. Bring to a simmer over medium heat, scraping up any browned pieces on the bottom of the pan. Cook for 5–7 minutes, or until the glaze thickens slightly.

Return the venison medallions to the pan and ladle the pomegranate glaze over them until coated.

Place the medallions on a serving plate, sprinkle with any residual glaze, and top with fresh pomegranate seeds if preferred.

Wild Salmon Curry with Fresh Turmeric

Prep Time: 10 minutes

Cook Time: 20 minutes

Serving Size: 1 filet (makes 4 servings)

(Per Fillet):

Calories: 380

Carbs: 20g

Sugar: 3g

Protein: 30g

Fat: 22g

- 4 (6-ounce) wild salmon filets
- 1 tablespoon coconut oil (or olive oil)
- 1 medium onion, finely chopped
- 2 cloves garlic, minced
- 1-inch piece of fresh turmeric, grated or 1 teaspoon ground turmeric
- 1-inch piece of fresh ginger, grated
- 1 can (14 ounces) coconut milk
- 1 cup diced tomatoes (fresh or canned)
- 1 tablespoon curry powder
- 1/2 teaspoon salt
- 1/4 teaspoon black pepper
- 1 cup fresh spinach (or kale)
- Fresh cilantro, chopped
- Cooked brown rice or quinoa

In a large pan, heat coconut oil over medium heat. Sauté the chopped onion until transparent, approximately 5 minutes. Stir in the minced garlic, turmeric, and ginger, and simmer for another 1-2 minutes, or until aromatic.

Pour in the coconut milk and the chopped tomatoes. Combine curry powder, salt, and black pepper. Bring to a slow simmer, stirring regularly, for 5 minutes.

Gently set the salmon filets in the pan, skin side down. Cover and boil for 8-10 minutes, or until the salmon is fully cooked and readily flaked with a fork.

In the last 2 minutes of simmering, mix in the fresh spinach (or kale) until wilted.

Remove from the heat and serve the fish curry over cooked brown rice or quinoa. Garnish with fresh cilantro.

Rabbit Stew with Medicinal Mushrooms

Prep Time: 15 minutes

Cook Time: 1 hour 30 minutes

Serving Size: 1 cup (makes 4 servings)

(Per Cup):

Calories: 250

Carbs: 15g

Sugar: 3g

Protein: 30g

Fat: 10g

- 2 pounds rabbit meat, cut into chunks
- 2 tablespoons olive oil
- 1 large onion, diced
- 3 cloves garlic, minced
- 4 cups low-sodium chicken or vegetable broth
- 2 cups carrots, sliced
- 2 cups celery, chopped
- 1 cup mushrooms (shiitake, maitake, or reishi), sliced
- 1 teaspoon dried thyme
- 1 teaspoon dried rosemary
- 1/2 teaspoon salt
- 1/4 teaspoon black pepper
- 1 bay leaf
- 1 tablespoon apple cider vinegar
- Fresh parsley, chopped (for garnish)

In a large saucepan or Dutch oven, heat the olive oil on medium-high. Add the rabbit pieces and fry on both sides until browned (5-7 minutes). Remove the rabbit from the saucepan and put it aside.

In the same saucepan, combine the chopped onion and garlic. Sauté for 3-4 minutes, until the onion is transparent.

Return the rabbit to the pot. Pour in the vegetable or chicken broth. Add carrots, celery, sliced mushrooms, thyme, rosemary, salt, black pepper, and a bay leaf. Bring to a boil.

Reduce the heat to low, cover, and let it cook for approximately an hour, or until the rabbit is soft and fully cooked.

If preferred, add apple cider vinegar before serving for extra flavor. Remove the bay leaf.

Transfer the stew to dishes and sprinkle with fresh parsley.

Grilled Octopus with Oregano and Olive Oil

Prep Time: 15 minutes

Cook Time: 25 minutes

Serving Size: 1 cup (makes 4 servings)

(Per Cup):

Calories: 250

Carbs: 2g

Sugar: 0g

Protein: 25g

Fat: 17g

2 pounds octopus (cleaned and tentacles separated)

1/4 cup olive oil

2 tablespoons fresh oregano or 1 tablespoon dried oregano

4 cloves garlic, minced

Juice of 1 lemon

1 teaspoon salt

1/2 teaspoon black pepper

Lemon wedges (for serving)

Fresh parsley, chopped

In a large mixing bowl, combine olive oil, oregano, minced garlic, lemon juice, salt, and black pepper.

Add the cleaned octopus to the bowl and toss to thoroughly coat in the marinade. Cover and chill for at least 1 hour, or up to 4 hours for optimal taste.

Set the grill to medium-high heat. If using a charcoal barbecue, make sure the coals are hot and ashy.

Remove the octopus from the marinade and let any excess drop out. Put the octopus straight on the grill. Grill for 3-4 minutes on each side, or until the tentacles are browned and tender, about 20 minutes total.

Remove the octopus from the grill and allow it to rest for a few minutes. Slice into bite-sized pieces and serve warm, topped with fresh parsley and lemon wedges.

.

Bison Bone Broth Bowl with Ginger

Prep Time: 15 minutes

Cook Time: 45 minutes

Serving Size: 1 bowl (makes 2 servings)

(Per Bowl):

Calories: 310

Carbs: 35g

Sugar: 4g

Protein: 15g

Fat: 10g

4 cups bison bone broth (store-bought or homemade)

1-inch piece of fresh ginger, sliced

1 cup sliced mushrooms (shiitake or cremini work well)

1 cup diced carrots

1 cup chopped kale or spinach

1/2 cup cooked brown rice or quinoa

2 green onions, sliced

2 tablespoons low-sodium soy sauce or tamari (for gluten-free)

1 tablespoon sesame oil (optional)

Salt and pepper to taste

Fresh cilantro or parsley for garnish

In a large saucepan, bring the bison bone broth to a simmer over medium heat. Allow the sliced ginger to infuse for about 10 minutes.

Stir in the sliced mushrooms, diced carrots, and chopped kale or spinach. Simmer for a further 15-20 minutes, or until the veggies are soft.

In the last few minutes of simmering, stir in the cooked brown rice or quinoa, as well as the low-sodium soy sauce or tamari. Stir well and let it cook through.

Add salt and pepper as required. If desired, sprinkle with sesame oil for added taste.

Ladle the soup into dishes and top with sliced green onions and fresh herbs, if preferred.

.

Steamed Clams with Saffron and Fennel

Prep Time: 10 minutes

Cook Time: 15 minutes

Serving Size: 1 cup (makes 4 servings)

(Per Cup):

Calories: 180

Carbs: 8g

Sugar: 1g

Protein: 20g

Fat: 7g

2 pounds fresh clams (such as littlenecks or steamers), cleaned and scrubbed

1 tablespoon olive oil

1 medium onion, finely chopped

1 bulb fennel, thinly sliced (reserve fronds for garnish)

2 cloves garlic, minced

1/2 teaspoon saffron threads

1 cup vegetable broth or white wine

1/2 teaspoon red pepper flakes

Salt and black pepper, to taste

Fresh lemon wedges (for serving)

Soak saffron threads in 2 teaspoons of warm water for around 5 minutes to unleash their taste and color.

To sauté the vegetables, heat olive oil in a big pot or deep pan over medium heat. Cook for approximately 5 minutes, until the onion and fennel are softened. Stir in the minced garlic and simmer for another minute.

Pour in the vegetable broth or white wine, then add the soaked saffron (with water), red pepper flakes (if using), salt, and black pepper. Heat the mixture to a simmer.

Place the cleaned clams into the saucepan. Cover and steam for 5–7 minutes, or until the clams open. Discard any clams that stay unopened.

Carefully place the clams and broth in serving cups. Garnish with the saved fennel fronds and serve with fresh lemon wedges..

Guinea Fowl with Sage and Apple Cider

Prep Time: 15 minutes

Cook Time: 1 hour

Serving Size: 1/4 bird (makes 4 servings)

(Per Serving):

Calories: 320

Carbs: 8g

Sugar: 4g

Protein: 32g

Fat: 18g

1 whole guinea fowl (about 3-4 pounds)

1 cup apple cider (unsweetened)

1 tablespoon fresh sage, chopped or 1 teaspoon dried sage

2 tablespoons olive oil

4 cloves garlic, minced

1 onion, quartered

2 cups baby spinach

Salt and pepper to taste

Fresh sage leaves for garnish

Set your oven to 375°F (190°C).

Rinse the guinea fowl in cold water and dry it with paper towels. Season both inside and exterior with salt and pepper.

In a small bowl, combine apple cider, sage, garlic, and olive oil. Pour some marinade inside the guinea fowl's cavity and brush the remainder over the skin.

Place the guinea chicken in a roasting pan, surrounded with quartered onions. Roast for approximately an hour in a preheated oven, or until the internal temperature reaches 165°F (75°C) and the juices are clear. Baste the chicken with pan juices halfway through cooking.

While the guinea fowl roasts, sauté the young spinach in a skillet with a little olive oil until wilted. Season with salt and pepper.

Once the guinea fowl is cooked, take it out of the oven and let it rest for 10 minutes before cutting. Serve with sautéed spinach and, if wanted, garnish with fresh sage leaves.

Pheasant with Juniper and Blackberries

Prep Time: 15 minutes

Cook Time: 35 minutes

Serving Size: 1 pheasant breast (makes 4 servings)

(Per Serving):

Calories: 240

Carbs: 8g

Sugar: 3g

Protein: 28g

Fat: 10g

4 pheasant breasts (or thighs)

1 tablespoon olive oil

1/2 teaspoon salt

1/4 teaspoon black pepper

1 tablespoon juniper berries, crushed

1 cup fresh blackberries (plus extra for garnish)

1/2 cup chicken or vegetable broth

2 tablespoons balsamic vinegar

Fresh thyme sprigs for garnish

Pat the pheasant breasts dry using paper towels, then season with salt, black pepper, and crushed juniper berries.

To sear the pheasant, heat olive oil in a large pan over medium-high heat. Add the pheasant breasts and sear for 5 minutes on each side, or until browned. Remove the pheasant from the skillet and put it aside.

In the same pan, sauté the blackberries for 2-3 minutes until softened. Add the broth and balsamic vinegar, scraping the bottom of the pan to deglaze and blend the flavors. Bring to a simmer.

Return the pheasant to the pan and place it in the blackberry sauce. Reduce the heat to low, cover, and simmer for an additional 15-20 minutes, or until the pheasant is well cooked.

Plate the pheasant and ladle the blackberry sauce on top. If preferred, garnish with more blackberries and fresh thyme sprigs..

Monkfish Liver Pâté with Green Tea

Prep Time: 15 minutes

Cook Time: 10 minutes

Serving Size: 2 tablespoons (makes about 8 servings)

(Per 2-Tablespoon Serving):

Calories: 100

Carbs: 4g

Sugar: 0g

Protein: 8g

Fat: 7g

- 1 cup monkfish liver (cleaned)
- 1 cup vegetable broth
- 1/4 cup brewed green tea (cooled)
- 1 tablespoon olive oil
- 1 teaspoon lemon juice
- 1/2 teaspoon garlic powder
- 1/4 teaspoon salt
- 1/4 teaspoon black pepper
- Fresh herbs (like chives or parsley) for garnish
- Whole grain crackers or toasted bread for serving

In a small saucepan, heat the vegetable broth to a simmer. Add the monkfish liver and gently poach for 5 minutes, or until cooked through. Remove from heat and let it cool slightly.

In a food processor, blend the poached monkfish liver with the brewed green tea, olive oil, lemon juice, garlic powder, salt, and black pepper. Blend until smooth and creamy.

Place the pâté in a serving dish, cover, and chill for at least 1 hour to enable the flavors to combine.

Garnish with fresh herbs, if preferred. Serve the pâté over whole grain crackers or toasted bread..

.

Elk Tenderloin with Wild Blueberry Sauce

Prep Time: 15 minutes

Cook Time: 20 minutes

Serving Size: 1 tenderloin (makes 4 servings)

(Per Serving):

Calories: 300

Carbs: 20g

Sugar: 10g

Protein: 34g

Fat: 12g

- 4 elk tenderloin steaks (about 6 ounces each)
- Salt and black pepper, to taste
- 2 tablespoons olive oil
- 1 cup wild blueberries (fresh or frozen)
- 1/4 cup balsamic vinegar
- 2 tablespoons honey or maple syrup
- 1 teaspoon fresh thyme or 1/2 teaspoon dried thyme
- 1 tablespoon lemon juice

Using paper towels, pat the tenderloin steaks dry. Season both sides liberally with salt and black pepper.

To sear the steaks, heat olive oil in a large pan over medium-high heat. Once heated, add the elk steaks and sear for 3-4 minutes each side for medium-rare, or until desired doneness. Remove the steaks from the pan and allow them to rest while you make the sauce.

In the same pan, combine the wild blueberries, balsamic vinegar, honey or maple syrup, thyme, and lemon juice. Cook, stirring gently, until the blueberries soften and the sauce thickens slightly, approximately 5-7 minutes.

Slice the elk tenderloin and place it on plates. Spoon the wild blueberry sauce onto the steaks.

If desired, garnish with more thyme leaves or fresh blueberries. Serve warm.

Grilled Sardines with Cilantro-Ginger Sauce

Prep Time: 10 minutes

Cook Time: 10 minutes

Serving Size: 2 sardines (makes 2 servings)

(Per Serving - 2 Sardines):

Calories: 220

Carbs: 4g

Sugar: 1g

Protein: 24g

Fat: 12g

4 whole sardines, cleaned and scaled

2 tablespoons olive oil

Salt and pepper, to taste

1/4 cup fresh cilantro, chopped

1 tablespoon fresh ginger, grated

1 tablespoon lime juice (about 1 lime)

1 clove garlic, minced

1 teaspoon honey or maple syrup

Preheat the grill for medium-high heat. Rinse the sardines in cold water and blot dry with paper towels. Brush olive oil over both sides of the sardines and season with salt and pepper.

In a small bowl, mix together the cilantro, ginger, lime juice, garlic, and honey (if using). Mix well to make a sauce.

Place the sardines on the grill and cook for approximately 4-5 minutes on each side, or until fully cooked and with excellent grill marks. Flip gently to prevent breaking the fish.

Remove the sardines from the grill and place them on a serving plate. Drizzle the cilantro and ginger sauce over the sardines.

Serve warm, with optional extra cilantro and lime wedges on the side.

Turkey Heart Skewers with Turmeric Marinade

Prep Time: 15 minutes

Cook Time: 10 minutes

Serving Size: 2 skewers (makes 4 servings)

(Per Skewer):

Calories: 150

Carbs: 2g

Sugar: 0g

Protein: 25g

Fat: 5g

1 pound turkey hearts, cleaned and trimmed

2 tablespoons olive oil

1 tablespoon turmeric powder

1 tablespoon lemon juice

1 teaspoon garlic powder

1 teaspoon ground cumin

1/2 teaspoon salt

1/4 teaspoon black pepper

Fresh parsley or cilantro, for garnish

Lemon wedges, for serving

In a mixing bowl, add olive oil, turmeric powder, lemon juice, garlic powder, cumin, salt, and black pepper until well blended.

Place the cleaned turkey hearts in the marinade, making sure they are completely covered. Allow them to marinade for at least 15 minutes (up to an hour in the refrigerator for added flavor).

Set a grill or pan over medium-high heat.

Thread the marinated turkey hearts onto skewers, allowing a little gap b

Grill or cook the skewers for 8-10 minutes, rotating regularly, until well cooked and slightly browned.

Remove off the grill and let it rest for a minute. Garnish with fresh parsley or cilantro, and serve with lemon wedges as preferred.

GRAINS AND LEGUMES

Amaranth & Red Lentil Buddha Bowl

Prep Time: 10 minutes

Cook Time: 25 minutes

Serving Size: 1 bowl (makes 2 servings)

(Per Bowl):

Calories: 420

Carbs: 50g

Sugar: 3g

Protein: 16g

Fat: 16g

1/2 cup amaranth

1/2 cup red lentils

2 cups water or low-sodium vegetable broth

1/2 cup diced cucumbers

1/2 cup cherry tomatoes, halved

1/2 avocado, sliced

1 cup steamed spinach or kale

2 tablespoons tahini

1 tablespoon lemon juice

1 tablespoon olive oil

1 teaspoon turmeric powder

1/4 teaspoon salt

1/4 teaspoon black pepper

Fresh parsley or cilantro for garnish

In a medium saucepan, mix the amaranth with 1 cup water or vegetable broth. Bring to a boil, then decrease heat to low, cover, and cook for 20 minutes, or until the amaranth is soft and the liquid has been absorbed.

In a separate pot, rinse the red lentils and add 1 cup of water or broth. Bring to a boil, then decrease heat and simmer for 15 minutes, or until soft.

While the amaranth and lentils simmer, cut the cucumbers, half the cherry tomatoes, and steam the spinach or kale.

In a small bowl, combine the tahini, lemon juice, olive oil, turmeric, salt, and pepper. Whisk until smooth.

Divide the cooked amaranth and lentils into two dishes. Top each with cucumbers, cherry tomatoes, cooked spinach or kale, and sliced avocado. Drizzle with tahini dressing.

Top with fresh parsley or cilantro and eat your Buddha bowl warm or at room temperature.

Teff Porridge with Black Chickpeas

Prep Time: 5 minutes

Cook Time: 15 minutes

Serving Size: 1 bowl (makes 2 servings)

(Per Bowl):

Calories: 320

Carbohydrates: 50g

Sugar: 5g

Protein: 13g

Fat: 8g

- 1 cup teff grains
- 3 cups water or low-sodium vegetable broth
- 1 cup cooked black chickpeas (canned or homemade)
- 1/2 teaspoon turmeric powder
- 1/2 teaspoon cinnamon
- 1/4 teaspoon salt
- 1 tablespoon maple syrup or honey (optional)
- 1 tablespoon almond butter or any nut butter
- Fresh fruit (like sliced bananas or berries) for topping
- Chopped nuts or seeds for garnish

In a medium saucepan, heat the water or vegetable broth until boiling. Combine the teff grains, turmeric powder, cinnamon, and salt. Reduce the heat to low, cover, and cook for 10-12 minutes, or until the teff is soft and the mixture has absorbed the majority of the liquid.

Stir in the cooked black chickpeas and simmer for another 2-3 minutes, or until well heated.

If desired, add maple syrup or honey to sweeten and almond butter to thicken.

Divide the porridge into two dishes and garnish with fresh fruit and chopped nuts or seeds, if desired

Millet-Buckwheat Kitchari

Prep Time: 10 minutes

Cook Time: 30 minutes

Serving Size: 1 cup (makes 4 servings)

(Per Cup):

Calories: 220

Carbs: 38g

Sugar: 2g

Protein: 6g

Fat: 5g

- 1/2 cup millet
- 1/2 cup buckwheat groats
- 1 tablespoon coconut oil or ghee
- 1 teaspoon cumin seeds
- 1 teaspoon mustard seeds
- 1 teaspoon turmeric powder
- 1/2 teaspoon ginger (freshly grated or powdered)
- 1/4 teaspoon salt (adjust to taste)
- 4 cups water or low-sodium vegetable broth
- 1 cup mixed vegetables (e.g. carrots, peas, spinach)
- Fresh cilantro for garnish
- Lemon wedges for serving

In a fine-mesh strainer, rinse the millet and buckwheat in cold water until the water is clear. Drain and put aside.

In a big saucepan, heat the coconut oil on medium heat. Sauté cumin and mustard seeds for approximately 30 seconds, or until they pop.

Mix in the washed millet and buckwheat, turmeric powder, ginger, and salt. Pour in the water or veggie broth and heat to a boil.

Reduce the heat to low, cover, and cook for about 20 minutes, stirring regularly. After 15 minutes, add the mixed veggies and continue cooking until the grains are soft and the liquid has been absorbed.

Remove from heat and allow it to rest for a few minutes. Fluff the kitchari with a fork before serving warm. Garnish with fresh cilantro and lemon wedges if preferred.

.

Sorghum & Adzuki Bean Stew

Prep Time: 10 minutes

Cook Time: 40 minutes

Serving Size: 1 cup (makes 4 servings)

(Per Cup):

Calories: 220

Carbs: 40g

Sugar: 3g

Protein: 10g

Fat: 5g

- 1 cup sorghum, rinsed and drained
- 4 cups vegetable broth (low-sodium)
- 1 can (15 oz) adzuki beans, drained and rinsed
- 1 medium onion, diced
- 2 cloves garlic, minced
- 2 medium carrots, diced
- 1 medium zucchini, diced
- 1 teaspoon ground cumin
- 1 teaspoon smoked paprika
- 1/2 teaspoon turmeric powder
- 1/2 teaspoon salt
- 1/4 teaspoon black pepper
- 2 tablespoons olive oil
- Fresh parsley or cilantro for garnish

In a medium saucepan, mix the washed sorghum with the vegetable broth. Bring to a boil, then lower to a low heat, cover, and cook for 30 minutes, or until the sorghum is soft but somewhat chewy.

To sauté the vegetables, heat olive oil in a large saucepan over medium heat. Sauté the chopped onion and garlic for 3-4 minutes, until the onion is transparent.

Stir in the chopped carrots and zucchini, then simmer for a further 5 minutes, stirring regularly.

Once the sorghum has cooked, add it to the saucepan with the adzuki beans, cumin, smoked paprika, turmeric, salt, and black pepper. Stir well to mix. If the stew is too thick, add a bit more vegetable broth until you get the required consistency.

Cook for a further 5-10 minutes to enable the flavors to combine.

Ladle the stew into dishes and top with fresh parsley or cilantro, if preferred.

Job's Tears & Green Lentil Salad

Prep Time: 15 minutes

Cook Time: 25 minutes

Serving Size: 1 cup (makes 4 servings)

(Per Serving):

Calories: 230

Carbs: 34g

Sugar: 3g

Protein: 8g

Fat: 8g

1 cup Job's tears (Coix seeds), rinsed

1 cup green lentils, rinsed

4 cups water

1 cup diced cucumbers

1 cup halved cherry tomatoes

1/2 cup red onion, finely chopped

1/2 cup fresh parsley, chopped

1/4 cup olive oil

2 tablespoons apple cider vinegar

1 teaspoon Dijon mustard

1/2 teaspoon salt

1/4 teaspoon black pepper

1/2 teaspoon garlic powder

In a medium saucepan, mix Job's tears and water. Bring to a boil, then decrease the heat and simmer for 25-30 minutes, or until tender. Drain the excess water and leave aside to cool. In a separate saucepan, simmer the green lentils in boiling water for 15-20 minutes, until cooked, then drain and chill.

In a small mixing bowl, blend olive oil, apple cider vinegar, Dijon mustard, salt, black pepper, and garlic powder until thoroughly mixed.

In a large mixing bowl, add cooked Job's tears, green lentils, chopped cucumbers, cherry tomatoes, red onion, and parsley. Drizzle the dressing over the salad and gently toss to mix.

Serve the salad immediately or chill for 30 minutes to enable the flavors to mingle. Enjoy it cold or at room temperature.

Spiced Red Bean and Sorghum Bowl

Prep Time: 10 minutes

Cook Time: 30 minutes

Serving Size: 1 bowl (makes 2 servings)

(Per Bowl):

Calories: 350

Carbohydrates: 60g

Sugar: 5g

Protein: 12g

Fat: 8g

1 cup sorghum

3 cups water or low-sodium vegetable broth

1 can (15 oz) red kidney beans, drained and rinsed

1 cup diced tomatoes (canned or fresh)

1/2 cup corn kernels (fresh or frozen)

1 tablespoon olive oil

1 teaspoon cumin

1/2 teaspoon smoked paprika

1/2 teaspoon garlic powder

1/2 teaspoon onion powder

1/4 teaspoon salt

1/4 teaspoon black pepper

Fresh cilantro or parsley, for garnish

Avocado slices, for topping

In a medium saucepan, heat the water or vegetable broth until boiling. Add the sorghum, decrease the heat to low, cover, and cook for 30 minutes, or until soft. Drain any surplus liquid as needed.

In a large skillet, heat the olive oil over medium heat. Mix in the chopped tomatoes, red kidney beans, corn, cumin, smoked paprika, garlic powder, onion powder, salt, and black pepper. Stir and simmer for approximately 5-7 minutes, or until well cooked and the flavors have mixed.

Divide the cooked sorghum into two bowls. Top each dish with the seasoned red bean mixture.

Sprinkle with fresh cilantro or parsley and, if preferred, add avocado slices.

Buckwheat Noodle Bowl with Edamame

Prep Time: 10 minutes

Cook Time: 10 minutes

Serving Size: 1 bowl (makes 2 servings)

6 ounces buckwheat noodles (soba noodles)

1 cup shelled edamame (fresh or frozen)

1 cup chopped bok choy or spinach

1/2 cup shredded carrots

1/4 cup sliced green onions

2 tablespoons low-sodium soy sauce or tamari

1 tablespoon sesame oil

1 teaspoon grated ginger

1 teaspoon garlic, minced

1 tablespoon sesame seeds (for garnish)

(Per Bowl):

Calories: 320

Carbs: 44g

Sugar: 3g

Protein: 15g

Fat: 10g

Heat water in a big saucepan until it boils. Cook the buckwheat noodles according to the package directions (typically 5-7 minutes). Add the edamame to the saucepan in the last 2-3 minutes of cooking. Drain and rinse with cold water.

To sauté the vegetables, heat sesame oil in a large pan over medium heat. Sauté minced garlic and grated ginger for approximately 1 minute, until aromatic. Chop bok choy or spinach and shred carrots. Cook for 2-3 minutes, until the veggies are barely soft.

In the pan with the sautéed veggies, combine the drained noodles and edamame. Add the soy sauce or tamari and stir everything together until heated through.

Divide the noodle mixture between two bowls. Garnish with chopped green onions and sesame seeds.

Teff and Split Pea Soup

Prep Time: 10 minutes

Cook Time: 30 minutes

Serving Size: 1 cup (makes 4 servings)

(Per Cup):

Calories: 210

Carbs: 35g

Sugar: 4g

Protein: 10g

Fat: 6g

1 cup split peas, rinsed	1 teaspoon cumin
1/2 cup teff grain	1/2 teaspoon salt
1 medium onion, chopped	1/4 teaspoon black pepper
2 cloves garlic, minced	2 tablespoons olive oil
2 medium carrots, diced	Fresh parsley, chopped (for garnish)
2 celery stalks, diced	
6 cups low-sodium vegetable broth	
1 teaspoon turmeric powder	

To sauté the vegetables, heat olive oil in a large saucepan over medium heat. Combine the diced onion, garlic, carrots, and celery. Sauté for 5-7 minutes, or until the veggies soften.

Stir in the washed split peas and teff grain, combining well with the sautéed veggies.

Pour in the veggie broth and season with turmeric, cumin, salt, and black pepper. Heat the mixture to a boil.

Reduce the heat to low, cover, and let it stew for approximately 25-30 minutes, or until the split peas are soft and the teff is done.

To get a creamier texture, use an immersion blender to puree some of the soup or transfer it to a blender and blend until smooth. Return to the pot and stir.

Transfer the soup to dishes and decorate with fresh parsley.

.

Green Lentil and Wild Rice Pilaf

Prep Time: 10 minutes

Cook Time: 30 minutes

Serving Size: 1 cup (makes 4 servings)

(Per Cup):

Calories: 230

Carbs: 40g

Sugar: 3g

Protein: 10g

Fat: 4g

1/2 cup wild rice

1/2 cup green lentils

3 cups vegetable broth or water

1 medium onion, diced

2 cloves garlic, minced

1 cup diced carrots

1 cup chopped celery

1 tablespoon olive oil

1 teaspoon dried thyme

1 teaspoon dried rosemary

1/2 teaspoon salt

1/4 teaspoon black pepper

Fresh parsley, chopped

Rinse the wild rice and green lentils in cold water until they are clear.

In a medium saucepan, mix the wild rice with 1 cup of vegetable broth or water. Bring to a boil, then lower to a low heat, cover, and cook for 40-45 minutes, or until tender. (If using pre-cooked or quick-cooking wild rice, follow the package directions.)

In a separate pot, add green lentils and 2 cups vegetable broth/water. Bring to a boil, then lower to a low heat, cover, and cook for 20-25 minutes, or until cooked. Drain any surplus liquid as needed.

To sauté the vegetables, heat olive oil in a large pan over medium heat. Combine the chopped onion, garlic, carrots, and celery. Sauté for 5–7 minutes, or until the veggies are soft.

When the wild rice and lentils have finished cooking, combine them with the sautéed veggies in the pan. Mix in the dried thyme, rosemary, salt, and black pepper. Mix well to blend and cook for another 2-3 minutes.

Divide the pilaf among four dishes, garnishing with fresh parsley as desired.

Millet Porridge with Berries

Prep Time: 5 minutes

Cook Time: 20 minutes

Serving Size: 1 cup (makes 2 servings)

(Per Cup):

Calories: 260

Carbs: 48g

Sugar: 8g

Protein: 8g

Fat: 6g

- 1 cup millet
- 3 cups water or unsweetened almond milk
- 1 tablespoon maple syrup or honey (optional)
- 1 teaspoon vanilla extract
- 1/2 teaspoon cinnamon
- 1 cup mixed berries (fresh or frozen)
- 1/4 cup chopped nuts (like almonds or walnuts) for topping
- A pinch of salt

Rinse the millet with cold water to remove any debris. Drain well.

In a medium saucepan, mix together rinsed millet, water or almond milk, and a teaspoon of salt. Bring to a boil over medium high heat. Once boiling, decrease the heat to low, cover, and cook for 15-20 minutes, or until the millet is soft and the liquid has been absorbed.

Once cooked, mix in maple syrup or honey (if using), vanilla extract, and cinnamon. Mix thoroughly.

Divide the millet porridge into two dishes. Garnish with mixed berries and chopped nuts..

SMOOTHIES, TEAS AND BEVERAGES

Tart Cherry and Ginger Root Recovery Smoothie

1 cup tart cherry juice (unsweetened)

1 inch fresh ginger root, peeled

1/2 cup frozen blueberries

1 tablespoon ground flaxseed

1/2 cup coconut water

1 small beet, peeled and chopped

Combine all ingredients in a blender

Blend until smooth.

Golden Fennel Tea

1 fennel bulb, sliced

2 cardamom pods, crushed

1 teaspoon turmeric powder

1/4 teaspoon black pepper

2 cups water

1 tablespoon honey (optional)

Bring water to boil in a small pot

Add all ingredients except honey

Simmer for 15 minutes

Strain and add honey if desired.

.

Purple Power Inflammation Fighter

1 cup purple cabbage, chopped

1 purple carrot

1 handful black grapes

1 tablespoon pomegranate seeds

1 cup coconut water

1/2 lemon, juiced

Small piece of fresh ginger

Juice all ingredients except coconut water

Mix with coconut water

Serve over ice

Rosemary-Sage Iced Tea

3 sprigs fresh rosemary

5 fresh sage leaves

2 cups boiling water

1 tablespoon raw honey

1/2 lemon, sliced

Ice cubes

Steep herbs in boiling water for 10 minutes

Strain and let cool

Add honey and lemon

Serve over ice.

White Pine Needle and Blackberry Tea

2 tablespoons fresh white pine needles (from edible pine species only)

1/2 cup fresh blackberries

2 cups water

1 cinnamon stick

1 teaspoon raw honey (optional)

Bring water to a simmer

Add pine needles and cinnamon

Simmer for 20 minutes

Add crushed blackberries

Strain and sweeten if desired.

Nettle and Mint Elixir

2 tablespoons dried nettle leaves

Fresh mint leaves

1 tablespoon apple cider vinegar

2 cups water

1 teaspoon raw honey

Pinch of sea salt

Steep nettle and mint in hot water for 15 minutes

Add apple cider vinegar and salt

Strain and sweeten with honey

Serve hot or cold

Mushroom Anti-Inflammatory Latte

1 teaspoon reishi mushroom powder

1 teaspoon chaga mushroom powder

1 cup plant-based milk

1/2 teaspoon cinnamon

1/4 teaspoon vanilla extract

1 teaspoon MCT oil

Pinch of sea salt

Heat milk in a small pot

Whisk in all ingredients

Blend until frothy

Serve hot.

Evening Inflammation Relief Tea

1 tablespoon dried chamomile

1 tablespoon dried lemon balm

1 teaspoon dried rose petals

2 cups water

1/2 teaspoon vanilla extract

1 star anise pod

Bring water to boil

Add all ingredients

Steep for 10 minutes

Strain and serve.

Bromelain Boost Smoothie

1 cup fresh pineapple chunks

1/2 papaya, peeled and seeded

1 tablespoon fresh mint

1 thumb-sized piece of ginger

1/2 cup coconut water

1 tablespoon chia seeds

Ice cubes

Blend all ingredients until smooth

Add more coconut water if needed.

30 days meal plan

Week 1

Day 1
- Breakfast: Sweet Potato Hash (p.33)
- Lunch: Wild Salmon & Berry Salad (p.58)
- Dinner: Turmeric-Ginger Poached Sea Bass with Saffron Broth (p.143)
- Smoothie: Tart Cherry and Ginger Root Recovery Smoothie (p.200)

Day 2
- Breakfast: Overnight Oats (p.35)
- Lunch: Turmeric Roasted Cauliflower Salad (p.59)
- Dinner: Duck Breast with Tart Cherry Reduction (p.146)
- Tea: Golden Fennel Tea (p.201)

Day 3
- Breakfast: Ginger-Spiced Oatmeal (p.38)
- Lunch: Mediterranean Chickpea Bowl (p.68)
- Dinner: Brazilian Fish Stew (Moqueca) (p.127)
- Smoothie: Purple Power Inflammation Fighter (p.202)

Day 4
- Breakfast: Mediterranean Breakfast Plate (p.39)
- Lunch: Sweet Potato & Black Bean Buddha Bowl (p.69)
- Dinner: Black Cod Misoyaki with Wasabi Greens (p.156)
- Tea: Rosemary-Sage Iced Tea (p.203)

Day 5
- Breakfast: Berry-Loaded Quinoa Bowl (p.40)
- Lunch: Mediterranean Tuna Salad (p.79)
- Dinner: Rabbit Stew with Medicinal Mushrooms (p.162)
- Smoothie: Evening Inflammation Relief Tea (p.207)

Day 6
- Breakfast: Turmeric Potato Scramble (p.41)
- Lunch: Lentil & Roasted Vegetable Bowl (p.72)

- Dinner: Ethiopian Red Lentil Stew (Misir Wat) (p.138)
- Smoothie: Bromelain Boost Smoothie (p.208)

Day 7
- Breakfast: Cinnamon Apple Oatmeal (p.43)
- Lunch: Roasted Vegetable & Quinoa Bowl (p.75)
- Dinner: Grilled Octopus with Oregano and Olive Oil (p.164)
- Tea: White Pine Needle and Blackberry Tea (p.204)

Week 2

Day 8
- Breakfast: Potato Breakfast Bowl (p.37)
- Lunch: Greek Kale Bowl (p.61)
- Dinner: Mackerel En Papillote with Green Tea and Citrus (p.144)
- Tea: Nettle and Mint Elixir (p.205)

Day 9
- Breakfast: Toast (p.42)
- Lunch: Mediterranean Hummus Wrap (p.63)
- Dinner: Venison Medallions with Pomegranate Glaze (p.158)
- Smoothie: Tart Cherry and Ginger Root Recovery Smoothie (p.200)

Day 10
- Breakfast: Sweet Potato Toast (p.44)
- Lunch: Rainbow Poke Bowl (p.70)
- Dinner: Grilled Sardines with Cilantro-Ginger Sauce (p.177)
- Tea: Golden Fennel Tea (p.201)

Day 11
- Breakfast: Quick Chia Pudding (p.47)
- Lunch: Greek Shrimp Salad (p.74)
- Dinner: Bison Bone Broth Bowl with Ginger (p.166)
- Smoothie: Purple Power Inflammation Fighter (p.202)

Day 12
- Breakfast: Savory Oatmeal Bowl (p.48)
- Lunch: Mediterranean Quinoa Bowl (p.56)

- Dinner: Broiled Quail with Green Tea Rub (p.154)
- Tea: Rosemary-Sage Iced Tea (p.203)

Day 13
- Breakfast: Potato and Egg Muffins (p.45)
- Lunch: Collard Green Turkey Wrap (p.62)
- Dinner: Thai Coconut Kabocha Squash Soup (p.134)
- Smoothie: Evening Inflammation Relief Tea (p.207)

Day 14
- Breakfast: Quick Apple-Carrot Oats (p.53)
- Lunch: Miso Glazed Tofu Bowl (p.82)
- Dinner: Guinea Fowl with Sage and Apple Cider (p.170)
- Smoothie: Bromelain Boost Smoothie (p.208)

Week 3

Day 15
- Breakfast: Sheet Pan Breakfast (p.54)
- Lunch: Grilled Chicken & Avocado Lettuce Cups (p.80)
- Dinner: Sardine and Anchovy Puttanesca (p.148)
- Tea: Mushroom Anti-Inflammatory Latte (p.206)

Day 16
- Breakfast: Rice Bowl (p.51)
- Lunch: Wild Rice & Cranberry Salad (p.78)
- Dinner: Golden Bone Broth Soup with Root Vegetables (p.131)
- Smoothie: Tart Cherry and Ginger Root Recovery Smoothie (p.200)

Day 17
- Breakfast: Sweet Potato Hash (p.33)
- Lunch: Greek Kale Bowl (p.61)
- Dinner: Monkfish Liver Pâté with Green Tea (p.174)
- Tea: Golden Fennel Tea (p.201)

Day 18
- Breakfast: Cinnamon Apple Oatmeal (p.43)
- Lunch: Greek Shrimp Salad (p.74)

- Dinner: Roasted Vegetable & Quinoa Bowl (p.75)
- Smoothie: Purple Power Inflammation Fighter (p.202)

Day 19
- Breakfast: Mediterranean Breakfast Plate (p.39)
- Lunch: Asian-Style Lettuce Wraps (p.64)
- Dinner: Grilled Octopus with Oregano and Olive Oil (p.164)
- Tea: Rosemary-Sage Iced Tea (p.203)

Day 20
- Breakfast: Turmeric Potato Scramble (p.41)
- Lunch: Sweet Potato & Black Bean Buddha Bowl (p.69)
- Dinner: Duck Breast with Tart Cherry Reduction (p.146)
- Smoothie: Evening Inflammation Relief Tea (p.207)

Day 21
- Breakfast: Toast (p.42)
- Lunch: Mediterranean Tuna Salad (p.79)
- Dinner: Persian Pomegranate Walnut Stew (Fesenjan) (p.133)
- Tea: White Pine Needle and Blackberry Tea (p.204)

Week 4

Day 22
- Breakfast: Berry-Loaded Quinoa Bowl (p.40)
- Lunch: Collard Green Turkey Wrap (p.62)
- Dinner: Grass-fed Liver with Rosemary and Blueberry Compote (p.152)
- Tea: Nettle and Mint Elixir (p.205)

Day 23
- Breakfast: Overnight Oats (p.35)
- Lunch: Roasted Vegetable & Quinoa Bowl (p.75)
- Dinner: Wild Salmon Curry with Fresh Turmeric (p.160)
- Smoothie: Tart Cherry and Ginger Root Recovery Smoothie (p.200)

Day 24
- Breakfast: Ginger-Spiced Oatmeal (p.38)
- Lunch: Rainbow Poke Bowl (p.70)

- Dinner: Mussels in Golden Milk Broth (p.150)
- Tea: Golden Fennel Tea (p.201)

Day 25
- Breakfast: Sweet Potato Toast (p.44)
- Lunch: Greek Kale Bowl (p.61)
- Dinner: Bison Bone Broth Bowl with Ginger (p.166)
- Smoothie: Purple Power Inflammation Fighter (p.202)

Day 26
- Breakfast: Potato Breakfast Bowl (p.37)
- Lunch: Mediterranean Hummus Wrap (p.63)
- Dinner: Broiled Quail with Green Tea Rub (p.154)
- Tea: Rosemary-Sage Iced Tea (p.203)

Day 27
- Breakfast: Quick Chia Pudding (p.47)
- Lunch: Mediterranean Chickpea Bowl (p.68)
- Dinner: Pheasant with Juniper and Blackberries (p.172)
- Smoothie: Evening Inflammation Relief Tea (p.207)

Day 28
- Breakfast: Roasted Potato Tacos (p.49)
- Lunch: Grilled Chicken & Avocado Lettuce Cups (p.80)
- Dinner: Ethiopian Red Lentil Stew (Misir Wat) (p.138)
- Tea: White Pine Needle and Blackberry Tea (p.204)

Day 29
- Breakfast: Sweet Potato Hash (p.33)
- Lunch: Miso Glazed Tofu Bowl (p.82)
- Dinner: Venison Medallions with Pomegranate Glaze (p.158)
- Smoothie: Tart Cherry and Ginger Root Recovery Smoothie (p.200)

Day 30
- Breakfast: Quick Apple-Carrot Oats (p.53)
- Lunch: Mediterranean Quinoa Bowl (p.56)
- Dinner: Persian Pomegranate Walnut Stew (Fesenjan) (p.133)
- Tea: White Pine Needle and Blackberry Tea (p.204)

Food elimination Meal Plan

1. Elimination Phase (Weeks 1–2): This phase focuses on removing common inflammatory triggers like gluten, dairy, soy, eggs, nuts, seeds, nightshades, added sugars, processed foods, caffeine, and alcohol. Meals will be based on safe foods, such as vegetables (except nightshades), certain grains, lean proteins, and low-glycemic fruits.

2. Reintroduction Phase (Weeks 3–4): In this phase, we'll gradually reintroduce eliminated foods one by one every two to three days. By observing any symptoms or reactions, it becomes easier to pinpoint specific triggers.

Elimination Diet Meal Plan: Weeks 1–2

Foods to Include:
- Vegetables (excluding nightshades like tomatoes, peppers, eggplants, and potatoes)
- Leafy greens (kale, spinach, arugula, etc.)
- Certain grains (quinoa, millet, amaranth, teff)
- Lean proteins (wild-caught fish, organic turkey and chicken, certain legumes)
- Healthy fats (avocado, olive oil)
- Low-glycemic fruits (berries, apples)

Foods to Avoid:
- Dairy, gluten, eggs, soy, nuts, seeds, nightshades, alcohol, caffeine, added sugar, processed foods

Week 1

Day 1
- Breakfast: Ginger-Spiced Oatmeal (p.38)
- Lunch: Wild Salmon & Berry Salad (p.58)
- Dinner: Miso Mushroom & Kelp Soup (p.125)

Day 2
- Breakfast: Sweet Potato Hash (p.33)
- Lunch: Collard Green Turkey Wrap (p.62)
- Dinner: Moroccan Harissa Lentil Stew (p.123)

Day 3
- Breakfast: Overnight Oats (p.35)
- Lunch: Turmeric Roasted Cauliflower Salad (p.59)
- Dinner: Grilled Chicken & Avocado Lettuce Cups (p.80)

Day 4
- Breakfast: Berry-Loaded Quinoa Bowl (p.40)
- Lunch: Mediterranean Chickpea Bowl (p.68)
- Dinner: Black Sesame & Purple Sweet Potato Stew (p.136)

Day 5
- Breakfast: Turmeric Potato Scramble (p.41)
- Lunch: Lentil & Roasted Vegetable Bowl (p.72)
- Dinner: Green Detox Soup (p.129)

Day 6
- Breakfast: Quick Chia Pudding (p.47)
- Lunch: Sweet Potato & Black Bean Buddha Bowl (p.69)
- Dinner: Ethiopian Red Lentil Stew (Misir Wat) (p.138)

Day 7
- Breakfast: Savory Oatmeal Bowl (p.48)
- Lunch: Mediterranean Quinoa Bowl (p.56)
- Dinner: Thai Coconut Kabocha Squash Soup (p.134)

Week 2

Day 8
- Breakfast: Cinnamon Apple Oatmeal (p.43)
- Lunch: Greek Kale Bowl (p.61)
- Dinner: Golden Bone Broth Soup with Root Vegetables (p.131)

Day 9
- Breakfast: Sweet Potato Toast (p.44)
- Lunch: Asian-Style Lettuce Wraps (p.64)
- Dinner: Brazilian Fish Stew (Moqueca) (p.127)

Day 10
- Breakfast: Quick Apple-Carrot Oats (p.53)
- Lunch: Mediterranean Tuna Salad (p.79)
- Dinner: Japanese Ginger & Daikon Soup (p.140)

Day 11
- Breakfast: Roasted Potato Tacos (p.49)
- Lunch: Rainbow Poke Bowl (p.70)
- Dinner: Persian Pomegranate Walnut Stew (Fesenjan) (p.133)

Day 12
- Breakfast: Potato Breakfast Bowl (p.37)
- Lunch: Greek Shrimp Salad (p.74)
- Dinner: Beet & Goat Cheese Salad (p.81)

Day 13
- Breakfast: Rice Bowl (p.51)
- Lunch: Mediterranean Chickpea Bowl (p.68)
- Dinner: Black Cod Misoyaki with Wasabi Greens (p.156)

Day 14
- Breakfast: Toast (p.42)
- Lunch: Wild Rice & Cranberry Salad (p.78)
- Dinner: Roasted Vegetable & Quinoa Bowl (p.75)

Reintroduction Phase Meal Plan: Weeks 3–4

Reintroduction Guidelines
- Introduce one food group at a time, every 2–3 days, while observing for any symptoms
- Begin with foods that are generally less likely to trigger reactions, such as eggs and certain nuts, then reintroduce soy, nightshades, dairy, and gluten gradually.

Week 3

Day 15
- Breakfast: Quick Chia Pudding (p.47) + Reintroduce Eggs with Potato and Egg Muffins (p.45)
- Lunch: Greek Shrimp Salad (p.74)
- Dinner: Moroccan Harissa Lentil Stew (p.123)

Day 16
- Breakfast: Ginger-Spiced Oatmeal (p.38)
- Lunch: Sweet Potato & Black Bean Buddha Bowl (p.69)
- Dinner: Black Cod Misoyaki with Wasabi Greens (p.156)

Day 17
- Breakfast: Berry-Loaded Quinoa Bowl (p.40)
- Lunch: Turmeric Roasted Cauliflower Salad (p.59)
- Dinner: Venison Medallions with Pomegranate Glaze (p.158)

Day 18
- Breakfast: Savory Oatmeal Bowl (p.48)
- Lunch: Collard Green Turkey Wrap (p.62)
- Dinner: Thai Coconut Kabocha Squash Soup (p.134)

Day 19
- Breakfast: Quick Apple-Carrot Oats (p.53)
- Lunch: Mediterranean Quinoa Bowl (p.56) + **Reintroduce Nuts** with pistachios
- Dinner: Grilled Sardines with Cilantro-Ginger Sauce (p.177)

Day 20
- Breakfast: Sweet Potato Toast (p.44)
- Lunch: Asian-Style Lettuce Wraps (p.64)
- Dinner: Green Detox Soup (p.129)

Day 21
- Breakfast: Cinnamon Apple Oatmeal (p.43)
- Lunch: Mediterranean Chickpea Bowl (p.68)
- Dinner: Golden Bone Broth Soup with Root Vegetables (p.131)

Week 4

Continue reintroducing in this order: soy, nightshades (like tomatoes, peppers, and potatoes), dairy, and then gluten. Each reintroduction should be made in small quantities with at least a 2-day observation period.

Food Elimination Diet Flare Up Tracker

Week 1- Elimination Phase

DATE	MEAL(s)	FOODS ELIMINATED	ENERGY LEVEL (1-10)

COMMENTS

Week 1- Elimination Phase

DATE	MEAL(s)	FOODS ELIMINATED	ENERGY LEVEL (1-10)

COMMENTS

Week 1- Elimination Phase

DATE	MEAL(s)	FOODS ELIMINATED	ENERGY LEVEL (1-10)

COMMENTS

Week 1- Elimination Phase

DATE	MEAL(s)	FOODS ELIMINATED	ENERGY LEVEL (1-10)

COMMENTS

Week 1- Elimination Phase

DATE	MEAL(s)	FOODS ELIMINATED	ENERGY LEVEL (1-10)

COMMENTS

Week 1- Elimination Phase

DATE	MEAL(s)	FOODS ELIMINATED	ENERGY LEVEL (1-10)

COMMENTS

Week 1- Elimination Phase

DATE	MEAL(s)	FOODS ELIMINATED	ENERGY LEVEL (1-10)

COMMENTS

Week 1- Elimination Phase

DATE	MEAL(s)	FOODS ELIMINATED	ENERGY LEVEL (1-10)

COMMENTS

REINTRODUCTION PHASE

Week 2- Reintroduction Phase

DATE	MEAL(s)	FOODS REINTRODUCED	REACTION TIME (IMMEDIATE/DELAYED)

COMMENTS

Week 2- Reintroduction Phase

DATE	MEAL(s)	FOODS REINTRODUCED	REACTION TIME (IMMEDIATE/DELAYED)

COMMENTS

Week 2- Reintroduction Phase

DATE	MEAL(s)	FOODS REINTRODUCED	REACTION TIME (IMMEDIATE/DELAYED)

COMMENTS

Week 2- Reintroduction Phase

DATE	MEAL(s)	FOODS REINTRODUCED	REACTION TIME (IMMEDIATE/DELAYED)

COMMENTS

Week 2- Reintroduction Phase

DATE	MEAL(s)	FOODS REINTRODUCED	REACTION TIME (IMMEDIATE/DELAYED)

COMMENTS

Week 2- Reintroduction Phase

DATE	MEAL(s)	FOODS REINTRODUCED	REACTION TIME (IMMEDIATE/DELAYED)

COMMENTS

Week 2- Reintroduction Phase

DATE	MEAL(s)	FOODS REINTRODUCED	REACTION TIME (IMMEDIATE/DELAYED)

COMMENTS

Week 2- Reintroduction Phase

DATE	MEAL(s)	FOODS REINTRODUCED	REACTION TIME (IMMEDIATE/DELAYED)

COMMENTS

Week 2- Reintroduction Phase

DATE	MEAL(s)	FOODS REINTRODUCED	REACTION TIME (IMMEDIATE/DELAYED)

COMMENTS

Week 2- Reintroduction Phase

DATE	MEAL(s)	FOODS REINTRODUCED	REACTION TIME (IMMEDIATE/DELAYED)

COMMENTS

Week 2- Reintroduction Phase

DATE	MEAL(s)	FOODS REINTRODUCED	REACTION TIME (IMMEDIATE/DELAYED)

COMMENTS